WITHDRAWN

P9-CCV-024

616.047 MIN
Living beyond pain : a holisti

"Opioids are killing more Americans than war or crime. We know the problem, but is there a solution? After all, the reason a lot of Americans take opioids is to deal with real pain. It's just that the 'cure' has become worse than the malady! Dr. Linda Mintle and Dr. James Kribs have teamed up to help people cope with pain without addiction to opioids by using clinically tested alternatives. Some books about opioids sound the fire alarm. This one is the fire truck coming to put out the fire."

Mike Huckabee, governor of Arkansas, 1996–2007; host of *Huckabee* on TBN; Fox News contributor; bestselling author; speaker

"Our nation is being ravaged by opioid abuse. *Living beyond Pain* addresses alternative ways to manage chronic pain and avoid destructive opioid addiction. This is an essential resource at just the right time, educating sufferers and caregivers alike regarding how to deal with pain in healthy ways and move away from the tragic national impact of opioid abuse."

Benjamin S. Carson Sr., MD

"Pain is a part of the human condition and always will be, this side of heaven. Pain can drain us emotionally, physically, and spiritually. It can take us to the point where we are ready to give up on life completely. How can we get beyond the crippling effects of pain and move to a place of peace by learning to live with pain? This powerfully impacting and tender book will teach hurting people how to do just that. Don't give up! Learn how to walk through life with the companion of pain."

Janet Parshall, nationally syndicated talk show host, author

"The healing of any malady—pain not the least—will emerge for an individual in a deep and sustainable way only in the presence of profound empathy, helpful information, and practical intervention. With *Living beyond Pain*, Linda Mintle and James Kribs have given us all three. At a time when our society is drowning in the quicksand of pain with few comprehensive offerings to provide trustworthy assistance, this book arrives, providing hope and confidence that pain no longer has to be the primary author of your story. For the pain sufferer who longs to flourish rather than merely survive, I can think of no better place to start."

Curt Thompson, MD; psychiatrist; author, *The Soul of Shame* and *Anatomy of the Soul*

River Forest Public Library
735 Lathrop Avenue
River Forest, IL 60305
708-366-5205
October   2019

"Being a professional baseball player didn't make me immune from pain. From personal experience, I know all too well the need to help people off opioids yet still manage their pain. These authors are the real deal. They know what they are talking about and can help you with your pain. It's a must-add to your personal library."

Darryl Strawberry, former MLB player, evangelist

"Our nation's military and veteran populations are highly impacted by America's ongoing opioid epidemic. These selfless servants experience high levels of trauma and injury resulting in chronic pain, particularly among our returning warriors who often need significant pain management measures during recovery and beyond. *Living beyond Pain* is a true gift to these warriors and their caregivers, training them to achieve effective pain management without the risk of devastating opioid addiction."

Robert F. Dees, retired major general, US Army; president, Resilience Consulting; author, *Resilience God Style*

"This fine work by experts outlining approaches to pain management is sure to help patients, families, and professionals confront the challenges of pain and implement effective evidence-based solutions that are well-established in the medical sciences and behavioral health."

Chad Brands, MD, pioneering hospitalist, academic health systems executive

"Physical, mental, and emotional pain are bad enough, but even more tragic is the devastation of addiction. As a former addict, I am committed to an all-out war against opioid addiction in America. I strongly endorse *Living beyond Pain*, a resource that provides healthy alternatives to the over-subscribed and dangerous opioids that put all of us at risk. We must eliminate this threat to Americans everywhere. There is a better way!"

Michael J. Lindell, inventor and CEO, MyPillow; founder, Lindell Recovery Network

"This book embraces the growing epidemic of people with legitimate chronic pain from a variety of medical causations. The authors offer a menu of solutions to ease the suffering of these patients who want help, not addiction."

Michael Lyles, MD

LIVING
beyond
PAIN

LIVING
beyond
PAIN

A HOLISTIC APPROACH TO MANAGE PAIN AND
GET YOUR LIFE BACK

Linda S. Mintle, PhD,
and James W. Kribs, DO

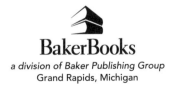

BakerBooks

a division of Baker Publishing Group
Grand Rapids, Michigan

© 2019 by Linda S. Mintle and James W. Kribs

Published by Baker Books
a division of Baker Publishing Group
PO Box 6287, Grand Rapids, MI 49516-6287
www.bakerbooks.com

Printed in the United States of America

All rights reserved. No part of this publication may be reproduced, stored in a retrieval system, or transmitted in any form or by any means—for example, electronic, photocopy, recording—without the prior written permission of the publisher. The only exception is brief quotations in printed reviews.

Library of Congress Cataloging-in-Publication Data
Names: Mintle, Linda, author.
Title: Living beyond pain : a holistic approach to manage pain and get your life
 back / Linda S. Mintle PhD, and James W. Kribs DO.
Description: Grand Rapids : Baker Books, a division of Baker Publishing Group,
 2019. | Includes bibliographical references.
Identifiers: LCCN 2019006892 | ISBN 9780801016776 (pbk.)
Subjects: LCSH: Chronic pain—Alternative treatment. | Chronic pain—
 Psychosomatic aspects. | Mind and body.
Classification: LCC RB127 .M57 2019 | DDC 616/.0472—dc23
LC record available at https://lccn.loc.gov/2019006892

Scripture quotations are from the Holy Bible, New International Version®. NIV®. Copyright © 1973, 1978, 1984, 2011 by Biblica, Inc.™ Used by permission of Zondervan. All rights reserved worldwide. www.zondervan.com. The "NIV" and "New International Version" are trademarks registered in the United States Patent and Trademark Office by Biblica, Inc.™

This book is not intended to take the place of advice of a trained professional. If you know or suspect you have a health problem, consult a health professional. The reader should regularly consult a physician in matters relating to his/her health and particularly with respect to any symptoms that may require diagnosis or medical attention. The authors and publisher specifically disclaim any liability, loss, or risk, personal or otherwise, that is incurred as a consequence, directly or indirectly, of the use and application of any of the content of this book.

Some of the names and details of the people and scenarios described in this book have been changed in order to ensure the individuals' privacy.

In keeping with biblical principles of creation stewardship, Baker Publishing Group advocates the responsible use of our natural resources. As a member of the Green Press Initiative, our company uses recycled paper when possible. The text paper of this book is composed in part of post-consumer waste.

19 20 21 22 23 24 25   7 6 5 4 3 2 1

We dedicate this book to all the people in pain we have seen in our thirty-nine combined years of clinical practice. We have heard your stories and listened to what it means to live with pain. We are humbled by your patience and transparency, are moved by your grit and determination, and hope to contribute to helping you and others live beyond pain. Those who are on the verge of giving up and fighting despair, don't give up. May you find hope, healing, help, and peace.

Contents

Introduction

Pain—A Part of Our Lives

Pain is no evil unless it conquers us.

Charles Kingsley

In a busy medical practice, clinicians often pause for a moment before entering a room to see a patient. It is a moment to catch their breath, collect their thoughts, and focus on what's important for the person they're about to see. In a clinic that helps people who are in pain, it is important to remember this before opening the door: the most effective treatment for pain begins with compassion and understanding. People want to be heard and understood. Their pain is real, and they need solutions. They don't want to be told not to worry or that the pain is all in their head.

Oftentimes, a patient will bring a spouse or loved one with them, and it is clear right away that even though one person is in pain, they both are suffering. This time was no different. A loving husband, John, was sitting with his wife, Clare, who had been debilitated by pain. "Doctor," he said, "she needs some relief. She's barely been sleeping, and I've never seen her this down. Honestly, it's hard to watch her hurt so much. It seems we've

11

done everything. What else can we do?" As I (James) glanced over at Clare, I saw a look of quiet resignation on her face. She was weary.

Everyone's story of how their pain began is unique, but there are common threads, whether an injury occurred or the pain came about gradually. When an injury or sickness occurred prior to this new life of chronic pain, the person recovered. They got better. Now they are experiencing something that doesn't go away. They can't get rid of it, and it feels as if they have lost control.

Pain has insidiously robbed them of even the smallest things in life. Perhaps they are unable to work. Perhaps they can't do their own shopping or laundry. Perhaps they can't play with their grandkids or be there for their spouse the way they used to be, emotionally, relationally, or physically. They may have had dozens of doctors' visits and have had to perpetually retell their story, all the while feeling cross-examined about how many pills they are taking, even needing to bring them in randomly to be counted or to pee in a cup. They didn't get to this place on their own, and now they are sitting in a doctor's office with guarded hope.

Clare and others like her are not alone in their need for help. Clare represents one of the one hundred million adults in the United States who suffer from chronic pain.[1] To put this in perspective, she is one out of ten Americans who experiences pain every day and has done so for at least three months.[2] In fact, chronic pain like Clare's is experienced more often than diabetes, heart disease, and cancer combined.[3]

Clare's husband, John, represents three out of four Americans who have personally witnessed pain in a close family member or friend.[4] Friends and family may not suffer physically, but they do struggle emotionally. They watch as their loved ones lose productivity at work, struggle to get out of bed, or sit in a chair, immobilized by a blinding headache. They feel helpless.

As a physician and a therapist, we are keenly aware that chronic pain is the leading cause of disability in America. However, pain reaches far past our borders and affects an astounding 1.5 billion people worldwide.[5] Pain is a universal experience, serious and costly.

Many, like Clare, have seen doctors for help. They are looking for a cure or relief, but pain is often difficult to treat, requiring digging and commitment to find solutions. For some, the reality of living with pain for the rest of their lives is not a message they want to hear. Still, pain can be managed and treated in ways that normalize life as much as possible. There is much that can be done.

John J. Bonica, an American anesthesiologist who is considered the father of modern pain management, defined pain as "a constellation of unpleasant sensory, perceptual, emotional, and mental experiences with associated autonomic, psychological, and behavioral responses provided by injury, potential injury, or acute disease."[6] In other words, pain is more than just an inconvenience for one's senses; it is a whole person experience that affects how a person perceives their body's function and how they respond to their world.

One way people may respond to pain is to become depressed. The stress caused by dealing with pain and its limiting effects may cause them to feel hopeless and helpless. The danger here is that negative emotions can amplify and prolong pain, which in turn further increases stress and depression. Thus, a formidable cycle ensues.

At the root of this is a loss of control. A person is no longer able to do the things they used to do. The loss is palpable. So how does one regain what was lost? From a medical perspective, the answer isn't as simple as prescribing pills, injecting a steroid into a joint, or providing a manual treatment. While what physicians provide can alleviate a certain measure of pain, a fifteen-minute office visit is often not enough to win against chronic pain.

Make no mistake, the pain isn't all in the person's head either. However, the way they *relate* to pain is entirely in their head. This is where the battle over chronic pain is ultimately won or lost. The battle is about optimizing their outlook and how they feel about and manage their pain. It is also about understanding pain itself and how and why it occurs. It is about understanding the pathways in the brain and in the body that have been altered as a result of pain and how to make strategic changes in life to affect those pathways in order to reduce pain.

Simply put, the better you understand pain, the better equipped you are to gain control over it. This is why we wrote this book. You can reduce your pain and resume your life. The process begins with compassionate care that allows you not to be embarrassed or to feel like a complainer. We've heard your stories and know your pain. We want to help make you aware of how to better deal with your pain.

As you read, you will learn more about all that contributes to pain. While your pain experience is unique, there are universal tools that can help. In the process of dealing with pain, you can move from hurting to hope to living again. You can take charge of your relationship with pain and find new ways to reduce and even eliminate pain. As we move through this journey together, you will find that living with pain doesn't have to define you. By the time you finish reading this book, your understanding of what causes pain and how pain is sensed in your body will have increased substantially. And the more you understand pain, the better your pain outcomes.

The approach we take is a holistic one, integrating the medical, structural, functional, emotional, spiritual, and social aspects of health and healing. Treatment of pain involves body, mind, and spirit and employs an interprofessional approach to treat the whole person. The physical, psychological, social, and spiritual parts of a person interact to perpetuate, worsen, or heal pain. Therefore, the whole person must be addressed.

Addressing all these parts of who you are is important to living beyond pain. While it may not be possible to remove all your pain, it is possible to have less pain and more function. Once you better understand how you can turn the volume up or down on pain, the more in control you will feel.

Through the strategies offered here, we hope you will better understand pain and find relief. We are excited to take you on this journey, knowing that at the end you will be able to live beyond your pain.

PART 1

UNDERSTANDING PAIN

1

Know Your Pain

Chronic pain is not all about the body, and it's not all about the brain—it's everything. Target everything. Take back your life.

Dr. Sean Mackey

At its most basic level, pain plays a protective role in our lives and is a normal response to injury or disease. Without the alarm system of pain, none of us would survive. It is when that alarm signal persists that pain becomes a chronic problem.

If you have seen a physician for pain, you have most likely completed a form that asks where your pain is, how long you've had it, if you had an injury, what makes it better or worse, how bad the pain is on a scale from 0 to 10, and whether it feels sharp, burning, numb, aching, or like an electric shock. Perhaps you've even been given markers and asked to draw your pain on an outline of a human form, front and back.

What is the point of all of this? First, your answers document the history of your pain. From a clinical standpoint, the better we understand how your pain started, the more accurately we can diagnose what is causing it. And just like anything else in medicine, the more precisely we can diagnose what the problem is, the more effectively we can treat it. Second, your answers draw for us a word picture of how you perceive your pain and start a dialogue to help us understand your pain. Your answers help us piece together the puzzle that needs to be solved.

Medical students have heard it said more than once that developing pattern recognition for the diagnosis of illness and disease is important. First, we understand what "normal" looks like. Next, we recognize something that falls out of pattern. Then we carefully analyze that information to make recommendations for treatment. For example, people who have diabetes, asthma, or gallbladder disease all have patterns we've learned to recognize. The more experienced we are, the more quickly we can recognize a problem when we see it and can differentiate that problem from what else it could be.

The same is true with pain. People who suffer migraine headaches present differently than those who have tension headaches or cluster headaches. People who have low-back arthritis present differently than those with a herniated disc, muscle spasm, or inflammation from overuse. So your physician should spend time getting to know you and getting to know your pain. Understanding the intensity, character, and quality of pain provides the opportunity to treat it more effectively.

Pain has generally been divided into three major categories: nociceptive, neuropathic, and inflammatory. Each of these types of pain looks different, and each of these types of pain requires a different type of treatment.

Nociceptive pain occurs when body tissues such as skin, fascia, muscles, joints, bones, and even internal organs are exposed to injury, or what your doctor would describe as a "noxious" event. Mechanical low-back pain is a type of nociceptive pain. With mechanical low-back pain, compressive forces between the small joints of adjacent spinal vertebrae are created by gravity, postural strain, or uneven muscle tension, among other things. This compressive force not only restricts movement in the small joints of the spine but also reduces blood flow in those tissues, reducing the oxygen content and nutritional supply. All of these factors lead to nociceptive pain. This type of pain is usually described as sharp, aching, or throbbing. The nociceptive pain response is usually acute, and if the injury or compressive forces resolve, the pain usually eventually goes away as well.

Neuropathic pain occurs when there is compromise within the somatosensory nervous system. More simply stated, neuropathic pain occurs when there is disease, compression, or an injury within sensory nerves. Diabetic neuropathy and shingles are both examples of neuropathic pain caused by a disease in which nerve function and sensation are altered because of the disease process. Carpal tunnel syndrome, sciatica, radicular neck or back pain, and certain types of headaches are also considered neuropathic pain syndromes. In these cases, the nerve problem is due to nerve compression or altered function of the nerves themselves instead of a disease process. This type of pain has its own pattern, too, and is often described as electric, shooting, burning, numbness, or tingling.

Another major category of pain is inflammatory pain. Inflammation is a typical response to tissue injury and is part of the body's natural response as the healing process is initiated. Inflammation causes tissue congestion, redness, heat, and pain in *response* to an injury or infection as the body tries to repair itself.

Think of inflammation as being on the repair side of tissue injury as opposed to the pain caused by the injury itself. A normal amount of inflammation is necessary as part of the healing process. For example, if you have a sprained ankle or a fractured wrist, inflammatory pain occurs as the healing process begins. Inflammation can also occur as a healing response to infection. For instance, nasal passages and sinuses may feel congested if you have a cold, soreness results from an infection in the throat, and piercing pain may be felt from a middle ear infection.

In addition to injury and infection, inflammation can also occur in the presence of an autoimmune disease. In these cases, the body mounts a misdirected inflammatory response against normal tissue. Such persistent inflammation causes tissue destruction to occur. Inflammatory bowel disease and rheumatoid arthritis are examples of autoimmune inflammatory diseases.

Other times inflammation can result from overuse, such as a strenuous, continual strain on the low back, shoulders, or knees. This type of pain comes and goes, and inflammation becomes worse with activity. This type of persistent inflammation can cause harm over time, and the tissue, joint, or bony structures may become compromised.

Again, inflammatory pain is a different type of pain pattern compared to nociceptive or neuropathic pain. When people experience inflammation, they often feel heat, tissue congestion, stiffness, and even loss of function as a result of the inflammatory process.

It is important to note that the lines are often blurred between the classifications of nociceptive, neuropathic, and inflammatory pain, and often there is overlap among them. Other pain disorders also exist that are more nuanced and difficult to classify, such as fibromyalgia, in which the cause of pain is probably multifactorial and only beginning to be understood. Cancer causes severe pain due to a tumor or cancerous process compressing, infiltrating, or harming internal organs, soft tissue, or bone. Because many types of pain generators may be involved, such pain is difficult to classify. As a result, cancer pain is often thought of as its own category of pain.

Psychogenic pain is another category of pain that is often misunderstood. Often, this type of pain is miscategorized as being all in one's head; however, this is not the case. Psychogenic pain has a physical origin, but the symptoms are influenced by complex psychological and emotional factors such as fear, depression, anxiety, and stress. Headaches, stomach pain, and back pain are examples of pain that can sometimes have psychogenic components.

As mentioned, certain treatment strategies work better for some types of pain than for others. For instance, some types of pain respond well to medical intervention, whereas other types of pain require manipulation, physical therapy, or rehabilitation. Still others require mind-body treatments.

Regardless of the type of pain, when pain becomes chronic, it has to be addressed on the mental, spiritual, and emotional levels as well as the physical. Too often, pain is treated purely from the pharmaceutical side of the equation. While many people respond well to medication and improve, addressing pain on only a physical level is often an incomplete approach when dealing with chronic pain.

How you relate to pain in the context of your life, emotions, and spirit as a whole is as much of a determinant for success as anything else. The difficulty on the medical side is often the constraints of a short office visit. Oftentimes, a physician can only scratch the surface of the emotional, spiritual, and mental side of pain. This is why an interprofessional approach that includes medical, psychological, and structural approaches is the future of pain treatment. It is also why we are writing this book.

2

The Toll of Chronic Pain

Take the first step in faith. You don't have to see the whole
staircase, just take the first step.

Dr. Martin Luther King Jr.

How would you feel if you experienced a house fire and no one
believed you? You try to convince others that you are not making
this up. You have video, smoke-filled clothing, ashes of destroyed
possessions, but people keep telling you it's all in your head. Your
house is fine, they say. Nothing is wrong.

People with chronic pain are constantly trying to convince others
that their house burned down. They want to be listened to, taken
seriously, and affirmed. What they experience is real. Renee's story
is all too typical of what a person with chronic pain endures.

I Am Not Making This Up

Renee was referred by her primary care doctor to see me (Linda)
for an evaluation. After repeated visits and tests, her physician

could not locate the source of her pain. Frustrated by her continued complaints, he suggested that her pain was all in her head and wanted me, a therapist, to evaluate her for that possibility. Renee had already been passed around to multiple doctors. She had repeated her story so many times that it sounded like a script from a play. "Why won't anyone take me seriously and get at the cause of my pain?" she said that day in my office. "My pain is real. It is causing me distress. Please listen to me. I am not making this up. I just want some relief or a plan of attack. Do you know how demeaning it feels to have doctors tell me they understand my pain and then assume it is all in my head?"

Like Renee, so many pain patients feel misunderstood while dealing with the uncertainty of pain. Often, they have no diagnosis and therefore no plan. They hurt and don't know why. Unfortunately, such patients can get the runaround from doctors who are too busy to really listen and take their complaints seriously enough to do what is necessary to get at the root of the problem. Often, this is due to the time limitations of a practicing physician. Our current approach to medicine works against a physician trying to do their job. Typically, they have to see patient after patient with very little time in the schedule to dig deeply. Most physicians would like to spend more quality time with their patients but have to fight a system that wants quick fixes and works against a patient-centered model of medicine. But with pain, time is necessary to figure out the cause and rule out a number of possibilities. For people like Renee, the uncertainty of not knowing what is wrong is extremely frustrating.

After evaluating Renee, I sent her to a physician who was able to take the time to listen, do a complete structural exam, review her labs and films, and genuinely care about her as a person with pain. The doctor was able to locate the source of her pain and the mechanics involved in its origin and devise a treatment plan. Renee returned to my office three weeks later delighted. She was actively working through her pain. She no longer felt misunderstood. Her pain helped reveal an unknown medical problem, and it now made sense to her. Most of all, she felt validated and listened to by a caring health professional who took the time to help her.

Even when a doctor can determine the original source of pain, as in Renee's case, doing so may not make the pain better. Pain can be like a nonstop alarm—impossible to tune out. You try to hang on and cope, not knowing what to do to stop the constant pain that is destroying your physical and emotional house.

In Roger's case, the source of his pain was never uncovered. He has a condition called chronic pain syndrome that has been difficult to treat. His pain has persisted for over a year, and depression has set in. Not only does he suffer physically but his wife also recently left him for another man.

When Roger talks about his life, he says that chronic pain has dramatically changed his life. He finds himself growing more anxious by the day and fighting to relieve the depression he now feels. Roger's protective system is working, thinking his body is in constant danger. But something is wrong in the way pain is being processed.

With help, Roger is making significant changes and reducing his pain. He now understands how his body, soul, and spirit are reacting to chronic pain and has learned how to turn down the volume on his pain. But getting to this point required an acknowledgment of loss followed by finding ways to rebuild his life.

When the House Burns Down

A fire alarm is tripped by the presence of smoke to alert you to the danger of a potential house fire; similarly, when your physical body experiences an injury or illness, the pain alarm is tripped for protection. With chronic pain, the alarm continues to misfire. You feel like your house is still on fire. For Alison Hodgson, a house on fire was a literal event, yet there is much we can learn from her story of loss that relates to pain.

Alison ended a typical day by getting the kids to bed and retiring for the night. One of the children was unsettled and ended up in the parents' bed, awakening Alison, who got up to use the bathroom and then decided to pull out her book light and do some reading. It was 4:39 a.m. Her husband stirred and thought something was burning. Alison assumed it was her book light about to burn out, but her husband, Paul, got up to check. As he made his way into the hall, the fire alarms began blaring.

Never really thinking their house was actually on fire, Paul entered the code and stopped the alarm. But then smoke thickened, and the alarm went off once again. This time he realized something was wrong, very wrong. The parents gathered up the kids and the family dog and made their way out of the house. Reality set in. Their house was on fire!

Watching the burning house, they had no idea that a random stranger had set a fire in their garage. The fire moved fast and burned the house to the ground. The family escaped in the nick of time with only the clothes on their backs. Their lives were forever changed.

Alison wrote about this life-changing event in her book, *The Pug List*,[1] and talks about life *after* . . . after the house became only a shell of itself and had to be rebuilt from the ashes.

When you have an injury, disease, or trauma, it is like a fire raging in your body. Everything changes, and life is not the same. Like Alison and her family, you have survived but must confront the reality of your life after—after the illness, injury, or source of the pain. Chronic pain is the after. The alarm continues to trip despite the lack of fire. It is in the after that you learn to rebuild from the ashes.

Pain as a Necessity

Pain is necessary to our human survival. It signals a problem that motivates an action. Yes, pain is unpleasant—at times, even intolerable—but pain is a warning signal of threat or danger. Pain tells us there is a problem. It is the alarm signaling the fire.

The alarm was a gift to Alison and her family. The blaring sound alerted them to real danger. Some have described the pain alarm as a gift. Coauthors Paul Brand and Philip Yancey in their book *The Gift of Pain*[2] make the point that a world without pain needs to be reconsidered. It would result in problematic consequences. It would be like living in a house on fire with no warning system to save lives.

Brand came to this conclusion based on his work as an orthopedic surgeon treating lepers in India. Lepers, he observed, feel no pain sensations and as a result are susceptible to injury and loss of limbs. Brand writes, "Silencing pain without considering its message is like disconnecting a ringing fire alarm to avoid receiving bad news."[3] Pain is needed and has value.

For those of us not on the front lines of leprosy treatment, thinking of pain as a gift might be difficult. In the best of circumstances, pain warns us that something isn't quite right. But pain is miserable, and it hurts. It is not a gift we ask for or desire to receive. However, the way we think about pain will influence its outcome. For now, try to embrace the idea that pain has value yet to be discovered. If you think of pain as nature's alarm system and chronic pain as a retripping of that alarm, which needs to be turned off or turned down, this will help you approach pain in a helpful way. Not all pain is bad, but pain that lingers into the after is where problems begin to occur.

One of the reasons it is difficult to think of pain as a gift is because when pain is present, it temporarily immobilizes us and gets in our way. We rely on it to do its job, but when it persists long after its utility, we want it gone. We feel it, yet there is no way to measure the intensity of our pain. There is no fancy test that can help us say, "Aha, there is the pain!" Whether sharp or dull, constant or intermittent, burning or aching, pain can be debilitating and involve loss.

With sickness or injury, we usually expect to get better or recover. However, chronic pain challenges this expectation. It lingers, and it can be depressing if we don't address it in healthy ways. It demands we give up things we hold dear or surrender to a new normal. When it persists, it can rob us of even the smallest things in life. Perhaps we can't open a jar of pickles, do our own shopping or laundry, or simply walk to the park. We can't be there for our spouse emotionally, relationally, or physically as before. Chronic pain demands our attention.

After the Fire, Take Inventory, Tear Down the Ruins, and Rebuild

It is difficult to overstate the extent to which pain can disrupt a person's life. While for some, pain represents a persistent, annoying distraction that interrupts the flow of the day, others find it decreases their capacity to function. Pain may affect walking or doing physical activities they used to enjoy, thus affecting overall well-being. The extra effort required to do normal things becomes fatiguing, so there is less energy and incentive to do once-enjoyable activities.

When pain becomes chronic, it invades our relationships, finances, identity, and more. It tries to overtake our lives and will succeed if we allow it to. It can be persistent. Pain, when persistent, creates distress and impairment and can negatively impact quality of life.

Chronic pain forces us to stop, to take inventory, and to focus on what is valuable in our lives. If we approach pain positively, it can make us better people and teach us. It can bring compassion for others and for ourselves. It can help us rebuild a life with renewed meaning and purpose. But before we can embrace pain and look to reduce it or end it, we have to take inventory of the losses that have come.

When Alison and her family stood before their burned-down home, they faced loss head-on. "Here is the thing about a house fire, or really any loss: before you can rebuild, you have to tear down the ruins, and you can't tear them down until you make an inventory. You need to record everything you have lost. You're required—spiritually, emotionally, and materially—to give a reckoning."[4]

If you are dealing with chronic pain, it's time to take inventory and record what has been lost. Then you can tear down the ruins and rebuild.

3

Take Inventory
to Rebuild the House

Ring the bells that can still ring. Forget your perfect offering.
There is a crack in everything. That is how the light gets in.

Leonard Cohen

At the root of persistent pain is a loss of control. You are no longer able to do the things you used to do, and the loss is palpable. It is like standing on the lawn of a burning house, knowing there is nothing you can do but watch it become rubble.

A loss of control takes many forms—the loss of things, functions, situations, health, expectations, and dreams. Life has changed. There is a new normal. But remember, you have survived and can grieve those losses and heal. As you take inventory of the loss, you can begin to rebuild using the concept of marginal gains that will be discussed soon. Small changes you make will result in big changes.

The question is, How do you rebuild after the loss? Physicians and therapists who treat pain know it isn't as simple as prescribing pills. It's much more complicated. But there are ways you can take back control and begin to rebuild even in the face of uncertainty.

Rebuild Enjoyment

Julia, a commodities manager, had been an avid recreational cyclist all her life. She used biking as an outlet to relieve the stress she faced every day, from the responsibility of managing multimillion-dollar accounts of other people's money, to the relatable challenges of keeping her twenty-four-year marriage vibrant, to nurturing and guiding her two growing children into the adult world. The more challenging the week, the longer the weekend ride. She used this time to refresh and process her life and emotions. She always felt better after she finished, and there were times when she felt cycling was all she had to sustain her.

Julia had experienced minor, nagging injuries before, as every cyclist does, but now she was experiencing something different. About two months earlier, she'd started noticing tenderness on the outside of her left hip. At first, she noticed it an hour or two after she rode. Then she started to notice it when she got up from sitting at her desk at work, and when she woke up in the morning. Over the next several months, the pain became increasingly worse. It kept her up at night, and she could not lie on her left side. Worse still, the pain became so intense that after ten minutes into a ride, she had to stop. Her family physician ordered hip X-rays, but her joints looked normal. Her physician prescribed anti-inflammatories, ordered six weeks of physical therapy, and even injected the painful area with a steroid, and still the pain persisted. Finally, her physician suggested she may need to find a new exercise. The inflammation and overuse were causing pain and making it too difficult for Julia to continue to ride. Inside, Julia was becoming desperate, worrying that she might have to give up the one thing she had for herself that made everything else make sense.

Whether this pain was ultimately temporary or permanent, Julia was losing something she enjoyed and used to relieve stress. Now that thing of enjoyment was causing pain. Pain is often associated with a loss of enjoyable activities and has to be reconciled in some way. In Julia's case, her love for cycling remained, and she had to grieve the loss. To begin to rebuild, Julia had to accept this loss for now and find new enjoyable ways to reduce stress. She had to discover a new normal.

If you have lost an activity you enjoy because of pain, grieve the loss and consider new ways to build enjoyment again. For example, could you find a new hobby or coach others around something you love but can no longer do? What else could you do that might be new and different? Finding new ways to enjoy life is one of the challenges.

Rebuild Work and Passion

Art had been an English teacher at a local high school for five years. He was a student favorite because of his ability to make literature come alive and to draw conclusions that applied to students' lives. He relished the privilege of helping students feel connected to the world in which they lived and had a passion for teaching. He also suffered from excruciating headaches.

Art's headaches began when he was fifteen years old. Over the years, those headaches had progressively worsened. Often, he had a low-level headache that felt as if someone was squeezing the circumference of his head. Once or twice a month he had what he called "whoppers." Every time they occurred, his symptoms started with nausea. Within the next half hour, it felt as if an ice pick were being jabbed in his eye, and he was out of commission. Bright lights and commotion were intolerable, and he had to go home and retreat to the silence of his dark bedroom. He tried several headache medications, and while some helped a bit, they also had side effects that, for him, made it difficult to teach.

Obviously, this pattern interfered with his work. His absenteeism had cost him the opportunity for promotion and increased responsibility. Because of his headaches, Art was also facing possible job loss. Not only would Art have to deal with the financial hardships involved with losing a job, but he would also have to deal with the loss of his passion, teaching. Pain was interfering with his life's work. The daily satisfaction of bringing literature alive in the classroom was being taken away by unrelenting pain. Financial hardship, coupled with a loss of a passion, was almost too much to bear.

To rebuild, Art had to find a new way to fulfill his passion for teaching while he pursued further solutions to effectively manage his pain. He decided to become an online professor. This way, he could teach the literature he loved but be in an environment he could control. His passion for both literature and teaching continued but in a new way.

If you are in a similar situation, think of ways you can do the things you love differently. It may take problem-solving, adjustments, or changing settings or schedules.

Rebuild Identity

As a pitcher on a softball team, Jessica experienced shoulder pain that became increasingly more difficult to manage. Eventually, her doctor recommended that she take a break from softball. Yet softball had been her life up until now. She was an athlete. Being told that she couldn't play ball robbed her of her identity.

When Jessica had to stop playing softball, she didn't know who she was. She called pain an identity robber. It was a thief, stealing her value and worth. If she wasn't an athlete, she didn't know how to define herself. It is not uncommon for athletes who are injured and sidelined to suffer a perceived loss of identity.

Now pain defined Jessica's life, telling her what she could and could not do. She could no longer play softball at the competitive level. Her social life changed, as she was ignored by the other players. She felt invisible to her friends. She couldn't go to practices and was eventually removed from the team roster. For the first time since the age of five, Jessica wasn't playing sports. Who was she?

The energy it took to fight her pain depleted her. She was confused and teetering on depression. Pain was eroding her sense of self and becoming the focus of her life. She was having difficulty separating herself from her accomplishments, and pain was stealing those accomplishments. Without them, she felt empty.

To rebuild, Jessica had to acknowledge that pain was a part of her current self, but it did not define her. Jessica had to find a way to reconnect with her body. Her body could still do other physical things, like swimming and walking. While she had lost aspects of herself, she could fight to hold on to others. She could spend more time with friends, reengage in more family activities, and develop other hobbies and interests. She had to learn to incorporate new beliefs, attitudes, and capabilities into a reconceptualization of self.

Identity is formed based on perceptions of self derived from culture and others. Jessica's positive sense of self prior to her pain was from an external source—her achievement in sports. She struggled to see her worth apart from athletic performance. To form a new identity, Jessica needed to have a new sense of empowerment. Pain was one part of her life, not her whole person. Her identity could be redefined, coming from an internal source of acceptance and peace.

There was more to Jessica than winning or losing a game. She was a person who played softball, not a softball player. She used to think sports were the most important part of her life. Without it, what else did she have? Now she was forced to ask, Who am I apart from sports? She was challenged with the question, Why have I given so much power to an external source to define myself? Chronic pain forced her to take inventory of her identity. She needed to redefine who she was related to changed circumstances.

We all have ways that we define ourselves, such as mother, lover, friend, coworker, and so on. Chronic pain can redefine us and create a loss of identity. You may wonder, *Who is the real me?* Pain may be taking up too much space in your identity. It may be interfering with your feelings of worth, security, and more. People will know you in a different way now. The question is, Who are you apart from your pain? Rebuilding involves not letting pain define you. You are more than a person with pain. You might be creative, inventive, good with finances, empathetic, or compassionate. Find those other parts of you and develop them. Take an art class, serve at a food bank, journal your thoughts, and discover new ways to challenge yourself.

Rebuild Function

Andy was diagnosed in his fifties with lumbar facet arthropathy, a degenerative process that involves the joints between his vertebrae. For five years, he had tried everything: anti-inflammatories, home stretches, physical therapy, and even injections in his back. Eventually, he had become nearly bedridden, finding temporary and marginal relief in opioid medications. He felt like he was a drain on the system and a burden to others. At times, he felt suicidal. Andy wanted a future but was having trouble seeing one.

Andy's life consisted of sitting in a chair in front of the TV. He looked at the clock, prayed for relief, and waited to take his next dose of pain medicine to get him through the next several hours. When asked what he would like for his life, he quickly said, "To mow my lawn again, to go to the grocery store alone, and to drive my car." But his pain and dependence on Percocet were preventing him from engaging in those daily activities. The chronic pain affected Andy's daily life and the quality of his life. His physical health, mental health, and social functioning were all impacted.

There is a strong correlation between chronic pain and reduced physical activity.[1] Walking, doing chores, participating in social activities, and maintaining an independent lifestyle are just a few areas affected. In many cases, people with chronic pain are not aware of their decreased level of activity and may even overestimate their functioning. This can result in less motivation for change because they believe the status quo is the best they can be. As a result, people like Andy end up on disability. They lose confidence in their ability to manage their future or even have one.

Chronic pain often affects the back, neck, and extremities, which impairs function. The lack of use of a body part can lead to atrophy, weakness, and loss of range of motion. When muscles aren't used, they grow weaker. The saying "Use it or lose it" applies. Things that are stuck don't feel good. And when a person doesn't move, circulation decreases, scar tissue forms, and pain increases. In the end, a lack of function results.

To move through the pain, opioid medications are often used, but these do not work to solve the problem of pain. Often, progressively higher doses become required to cover the same amount of pain, and a person becomes sleepy, less active, cognitively impaired, and lethargic. Before they know it, a person is overmedicated and not living the functional life they desire.

An important question to ask is, When does pain move from being a temporary setback to a lifelong condition? Part of the answer has to do with addressing the loss of function. Take inventory in terms of your functioning. What are you able to do, what is reasonable for you to do, and what are your goals? Focus on what can be restored rather than what has been lost. If you are uncertain, talk to your physician or health provider. Come up with a plan to increase your functioning slowly but surely. It may be getting out of your chair, making your bed, walking down a hallway. Whatever it is, begin to increase functioning in ways that are safe but will make you feel more productive.

Rebuild Relationships

Joy's pain began years ago, after the birth of her third child. Things were not easy for Joy and her husband, Ryan, early in their marriage.

Money was tight, he was finishing his MBA, and their three children arrived in stair-step fashion. During this time, Joy's mother was diagnosed with breast cancer, a battle she ultimately won, but it was a scary time for Joy's tight-knit family. In the midst of this, Joy began experiencing difficulty sleeping. She would often wake early in the morning and find herself unable to fall back asleep, and as a result, extreme fatigue began to settle in. She also began to experience headaches and noticed achiness and pain in her neck and shoulders, which became more widespread over time. Then she began to hurt all over and sometimes had strange creeping and crawling sensations in her arms and legs.

Joy's assessment was that she had become a burden to others. Instead of taking care of her family, they were taking care of her. It didn't feel right, and the guilt was overwhelming her. She found herself struggling with depression and anxiety. How would her family function if she couldn't get back on her feet and contribute her part? The more Joy's guilt took over, the more depressed she became. Her husband didn't know what to do. He felt helpless and told Joy his feelings. While she was grateful he talked to her, she felt even guiltier. She was another person he had to care for. She felt overwhelmed and had thoughts of suicide. She knew she would never follow through on such thoughts, but she continued to worry about the burden she was placing on her family.

When pain interferes with the basic duties of parenting or interpersonal relationships, we can easily feel we are being a burden to others. If we are not accustomed to being in a dependent position or needing care, guilt can take over. Asking for help or acknowledging that we can't do what we once were able to do is difficult. For some people, guilt leads to depression and even thoughts of suicide.

Joy needed help to reverse her thinking and move forward on a path to rebuild her relationships. Her constant complaints about her pain were causing her husband not only to feel helpless but also to grow weary. As he attended to his wife's complaints, he was unwittingly giving those complaints attention, which led to an increase in pain perception on his wife's part. Joy was locking herself into a sick role in which the secondary gain was attention. She didn't want this type of attention but was trapped in a cycle of dependence. The family was beginning to organize itself around Joy's pain, which helped no one in the family.

When chronic pain is part of a family's picture, family members must make adaptations and adjust to role changes related to the loss that comes with a lack of full functioning. Family members can get stuck in wanting things to go back to normal or focusing too much on what might have been if the pain event hadn't happened.

Family members often have to pick up the slack or do more to help the person in pain. These role changes can redefine family relationships and need to take place with care and goals in mind or resentment and anger can result. Often, the one compromised by pain feels guilty, and the family feels helpless. This dynamic can be changed when the pain is better understood and dealt with in ways that lessen the burden. Finding a balance between dependence and independence is important so that loved ones don't unintentionally enable the person with pain.

Relationships often become strained when chronic pain is involved and you don't function as you once did. You can get angry or depressed or feel a host of emotions, but it is better to talk to those involved and find a new rhythm to function together. Your children and spouse need an understanding of your pain and how you intend to handle it. Withdrawing or staying silent will cause them to feel estranged from you. On the other hand, you don't want to share so much that your pain becomes the center of your relationships or overwhelms those you love.

You don't want your pain to become the focus of your attention and your family's life. Be clear about your needs and expectations, but don't fixate on your pain. Rebuilding relationships requires finding a balance.

Rebuild Intimacy

Jack and Ginger had been married for ten years. They described their relationship as loving and intimate. Physically, they enjoyed sex and felt this part of their relationship was always strong and satisfying. But chronic pain had changed that report. Ginger was having debilitating migraines, which at times were triggered by orgasms. She was now physically uncomfortable with intercourse because of her pain.

The couple was suffering, but they were uncomfortable talking about the situation. Their response was to avoid sex altogether. Jack didn't want to trigger his wife's pain, and Ginger couldn't concentrate on sex because of the fear that it would bring on a migraine. Chronic pain was affecting their intimacy. To rebuild, they needed to talk about the importance of sex and intimacy in their relationship and find ways to work around the pain.

Intimacy is a human desire and integral to a sense of self. We all need to feel loved and to give love to others. We are hardwired for human connection. Our relationships and sexual satisfaction matter and are important to our quality of life. Chronic pain disrupts intimacy and sexual expression due to physical limitations, feelings of depression, lack of energy, alterations in self-image, and the response of one's significant other.

Your pain itself can interfere with sexual intimacy. When you hurt, sex is less likely. The way you respond to your pain is also a factor. It's difficult to focus on intimacy when your attention is on pain.

Even when pain is managed, the side effects of medications can limit your sexual experience. Medications can diminish your sex drive, inhibit sexual function due to changes in your nervous system, and affect your blood flow and hormones, all of which are a part of the sexual response. While sex is meant to bring satisfaction and release, it can be hampered by embarrassment, pain, and frustration. A discussion with your physician about the side effects of any medication you take needs to be part of pain management.

Pain can create isolation and move you further away from your spouse if you allow this to happen. This emotional distance can ruin your relationship if it is not noticed and addressed. Even the strongest relationship can be challenged by chronic pain. Therefore, you need to make an effort not to let pain affect the intimacy of your relationship.

One area that you can control is communication. Honest communication with your spouse is necessary. But this isn't always easy. How do you tell your spouse that a certain type of touch is painful? Still, discussing what you need regarding intimacy is crucial. Yes, you might be hesitant to bring up sex, but a commitment to communication will help you rebuild the intimacy that might have been eroding due to the interference of pain. In some cases, you may need to see a couple's therapist for help to rebuild intimacy.

Rebuild Dreams and Expectations

Sarah always dreamed of becoming a world traveler. At a young age, she was fascinated with other cultures and pictures from *National Geographic* magazine. After high school, she became a flight attendant for a major international airline. Her job began to take her around the world, and she was living her dream.

One morning she was rushing to meet the crew in her hotel when she fell and fractured her metatarsal bone and sprained her ankle. For weeks, she was on crutches but noticed that her foot was becoming swollen and red. It was also highly sensitive to touch and cold temperatures. She described the pain as shooting, stabbing, pins-and-needles, and basically unbearable. She was also experiencing numbness, so she headed back to the doctor. Sarah was diagnosed with complex regional pain syndrome. Treatment included a series of pain blocks and opioid medications to ease the pain. Sarah's travel career was over. She couldn't walk, much less work. Her dreams were dashed. Her love of travel was put on hold, and she had no idea what her next step would be.

To rebuild her dreams and expectations, Sarah needed to accept the loss of travel for now but not give up on the future. Treatment was ongoing and she was learning to live with pain. She joined a travel club and began to investigate jobs in the travel industry. Eventually, she may be able to take short trips or travel on a train, in which she could move around more.

Pain not only hurts in the physical realm but also can destroy your dreams and expectations if you let it. It's easy to feel cheated, sad, disappointed, or even bitter. The plans you had, the dreams for your future, and the possibilities you see may all be affected by the presence of pain. You may be angry at the fact that you are in poor health, depressed because of new limitations, and fatigued from the pain. Your pain may cause uncertainty about the future or disappointment when you try to re-create your prepain past. Maybe you are anticipating more losses in the future, and you dread experiencing grief again.

A repositioning needs to take place with chronic pain. Doing an inventory helps. What can you hold on to, and what do you need to release? You have choices to make. You can hold on tightly to what you thought should be your lot, or you can accept the reality of life and discover new dreams related to change. Closure to what once was usually means you have to grieve. You are a character in the story of your life. Chronic pain sometimes changes the story line, but you can rewrite the rest of your life's plot. You can have a positive story line in which grief is tackled and you meet the challenge of change. You can find new dreams and keep moving on with life.

Concentrate on what you can do and motivate yourself to do a little more. Find new hobbies, new interests, new dreams, new expectations. Be proactive. What can you adapt or modify to reclaim some of what was lost or to reach new or different goals? What can you do to see yourself in a new light? How can you use the brokenness of the now to create a brighter future?

In Japanese culture, there is a tradition called Kintsukuroi. It is the art of repairing pottery that has been broken using gold or silver lacquer. The potter sees the pottery piece as more beautiful because it has been broken. The repaired flaws become part of the design.

People with chronic pain are like broken pottery. Lost dreams and expectations may fall to pieces, creating cracks in the design. The brokenness of chronic pain forces us to look at the flaw in our thinking. We value wholeness, not cracks, but the Japanese, who practice the art of Kintsukuroi, see beauty in the broken. Do you see beauty in your brokenness? When you look at the dreams and expectations shattered on the floor, can you embrace what has happened and begin to rebuild? Can you see yourself as more beautiful than before?

Acknowledge your lost dreams and grieve those dreams. Incorporate the broken pieces into the design of your life. Doing so will help you rebuild to form something beautiful. You are capable of great things. Don't hide the breaking. You are not ruined or without value. Find the gold and repair the cracks so you can rebuild your dreams.

Rebuild Hope

Hannah was an impressive young woman. From an early age, she was involved in athletics. She loved to run and worked at becoming the best cross-country athlete she could be. A typical day would find her running ten to fifteen miles.

When Hannah was sixteen years old and a sophomore in high school, something changed. During her first meet, she noticed a sharp pain in her chest. She described it as a stitch in her side that just wouldn't go away. Because Hannah had a friend who had suffered from a collapsed lung, she decided to see her pediatrician. Nothing was found, but she was referred to a pulmonologist. He diagnosed her with a pulmonary bleb. She had a small collection of air between her lung and the outer surface of the lung. She was told to take ibuprofen and live with the pain.

To be certain, Hannah saw a cardiologist, who also told her she was fine. But Hannah was not fine. She was living with a high level of daily pain that she was trying to handle on her own. As much as Hannah tried to push through the pain, she couldn't do it and sought support. Her senior year she went to a clinic for a round of testing and was diagnosed with slipping rib syndrome. Her fate: steroid injection in the ribs and live with the pain.

For Hannah, pain became part of her identity, and fear began to creep into her life. She faced the temptation that comes with chronic pain—the temptation to give up and despair. She knew she was capable of doing more than the incapacitating pain was allowing. She decreased her reliance on ibuprofen and decided to push through the fear. Fear was keeping her from doing what she wanted to do, and she wasn't ready to give in to it.

Before leaving for college, she began seeing a physical therapist, who started to address her pain from a structural standpoint, and she began to have some relief. However, the pain returned after she left for school and stopped receiving treatment. That's when I (James) had the privilege of meeting her, and we resumed the structural work through monthly osteopathic manipulative treatments (OMTs). Again, things started to improve. Slowly, through paying attention to her body's cues, she was able to move forward to become more active. She wasn't reckless. Rather, she listened to how her body responded in order to reengage in life.

Uncertainty and a lack of understanding about what was occurring in her body could have made it easy for Hannah to lose hope. But with the encouragement of her family, church, and friends, and through the depth and strength of her faith, Hannah is conquering her pain. She doesn't live in fear, is overcoming her pain, and is able to do active things. Her road to triumph can be yours if you don't give up.

Hope and despair are two opposing emotions, and there is a struggle between them. All the moments of pain in day-to-day living can lead to hope or despair. Hope requires action and directional movement toward the future. It is not static. Hope focuses on recovery. It is seeing threads of light in a dark tunnel. Despair is shaped by pain, limitations, dependency, worry, and fear. Hopelessness is the end result of despair. It is the end of the process of giving up and losing a future perspective.

When you are dealing with chronic pain, the feelings of hope and despair can alternate. Hope may be present at the beginning and then wane as time goes by. If you give in completely to despair, you arrive at hopelessness. But if you hold on to hope, you can survive and even thrive during the most difficult days.

Rebuild Your Life

Living with chronic pain is a process of adjustment as you attempt to regain control in areas of your life that have felt so out of control. How you react to the changes involved with chronic pain will determine your future in significant ways.

Some of you are still in shock that you are in pain and having to deal with its consequences. Others of you are feeling hopeless and mourning an identity, a role, or a function that has been lost. Grieving is good in that it allows you to reflect on your losses so that you know where to rebuild. But it is important not to get stuck in the grief, to move to acceptance and reclaim your life once again. This is the time to take inventory, face the reality of loss, and begin to rebuild. You can find something beautiful in what has been broken. You can rebuild your life.

4

When Pain Doesn't Stop

I often wished that more people understood the invisible side of things. Even the people who seemed to understand, didn't really.

Jennifer Starzec

Now that you have taken inventory and are ready to rebuild, it is important to understand the science of pain. An explanation of how pain works in the body will help you see how complex chronic pain is and why it can be so difficult to manage. Once you understand this, you can gain an advantage over pain and the pathways in which it travels within the body. The more you understand, the more effectively you can make changes in order to take back control of your life.

The key idea to understand is that for optimal control of pain, you need to access and control the pain pathways in your body in as many strategic places as you can. So let's start from the beginning.

Pain Pathways

When tissue injury occurs in the body, it activates a process called nociception. Information about the injury travels in small nerve fibers to the spinal cord. Sometimes the body responds reflexively to this information, such as when you withdraw your hand from a hot iron or jerk back when you step on a sharp object.

Other times that information travels up to the brain, which assigns to that message the sensation of pain. The feeling of pain is not registered in the body but rather in the brain. Here pain is assigned its location within the body, the type and severity of the injury is assessed, and the context in which the event occurred is recorded. Emotions are attached to pain as well. All of this happens to create a learning process by which we understand that something is dangerous—and we try to avoid it in the future. Thus, the nociception pathways and the sensation of pain within the brain work together as a protective mechanism to prevent further and future injury.

The experience and the sensation of pain occur in the context of our lives and our histories. The protective process partly explains why the perception of pain varies greatly from person to person. Pain perception can also change within an individual over time. This is why emotions, expectations, perspectives, and attitudes can contribute to one's pain level. In short, there can be strong emotions and upsetting memories attached to pain that may need to be addressed. Those emotions, and how to manage them in order to manage pain, will be discussed later.

Nociceptive pathways are much like a complex highway system. They have multiple lanes, on- and off-ramps, forks in the road, times of increased activity, gates that might open or close, and even "traffic cops" that direct a nociceptive message along the way before it reaches the brain. If multiple gates along the highway are switched open, that message gets sent to the brain to be interpreted as pain.

In the 1960s, Ronald Melzack, a Canadian psychologist, and David Wall, a British neuroscientist, proposed the gate control theory of pain, which, though our understanding continues to evolve, has been generally accepted by the scientific community as to how we process noxious information in the body and recognize it as pain in the brain.

As already mentioned, when an injury occurs, information about the injury is transmitted from the injured tissue to the spinal cord and then travels up to the brain. However, along this pathway, the signal encounters nerve gates and must pass through these gates in order to reach the brain. These nerve gates are actually different types of nerves called neuromodulators. These nerve gates function to reduce or stop the nociceptive signal to keep it from reaching the brain, where it is recognized as pain. If the activity on the pathway to the brain is strong or persistent enough to overwhelm the gates, the gates are opened, and when the signal reaches the brain, it is sensed as pain. Sometimes these gates are open long after the offending stimulus is removed or the injured part of the body has healed. The pathway can also develop a maladaptive response, and the message is either always being transmitted or is transmitted more easily. In other words, it is like the pain messaging pathway is always switched on or more easily switched on. This process is called sensitization.

At the root of this process of sensitization is neuroplasticity. Neuroplasticity refers to adaptive changes within the brain and central nervous system. The brain can learn and adapt to new things. For instance, when a person learns to play the piano, new connections are made within the brain and become reinforced and more efficient with practice.

Neuroplasticity also means that the brain can learn and adapt in negative ways. This is the case with chronic pain. In this instance, pathways can be sensitized and become more efficient and proficient in signaling the message of pain. The more constant and persistent the signaling is along the highway, the more entrenched the signal of pain becomes. Emotions linked to the pain can become reinforced as well. At some points along the pathway, changes can even become permanent, and an otherwise short-term, acute pain event can become an entrenched chronic pain problem.

From Acute to Chronic Pain

According to the American Chronic Pain Association, acute pain is "pain of recent onset, transient, and usually from an identifiable cause."[1] For instance, a person experiences acute pain after spraining an ankle while playing basketball or after cutting a finger while preparing dinner. A person may have acute rib pain after suffering from a bout of bronchitis and persistent coughing or experience acute sinus pain when they are congested.

Many times acute pain is a symptom of the body's responses that contribute to the healing process. These include inflammation, muscle spasm, and even an autonomic response, known as the fight-or-flight response. While these are short-lived and natural responses designed to restore the body to baseline and normal functioning, sometimes they can cause mild and even severe pain, which may be momentary or last several weeks. Acute pain is typically self-limited; once the pain stimulus is resolved or healed, the pain stops.

Chronic pain is pain that lasts even after the injury has otherwise healed. The pain functions more like a disease than a symptom. The pain pathway and its modulators have changed. John J. Bonica explained that the pain signal continues to be triggered due to a persistent cause and stimulus.[2]

Over the course of three to six months, if recovery does not occur or if pain is not effectively treated, the body can develop a maladaptive response that can perpetuate and even exacerbate the problem anywhere, and even at multiple points, along the pathway.[3] In other words, the mechanisms in the central nervous system that turn down the volume on pain no longer function properly.

The injury that caused pain may no longer exist, and may have even healed, but the pathway that originally sent the pain message to the brain remains open and unopposed. The brain receives the message of pain even after the original stimulus no longer exists. When this happens, even ordinary touch and pressure can become a source of pain.

Why this happens to some people and not to others is not exactly known. Genetic and environmental factors related to stress may be involved. However sensitization develops, it is a major player in chronic pain. When chronic pain continues, it eventually rewires the central nervous system and causes changes in the brain and spinal cord.

Many of the reflexes that the body has to respond to pain can also be altered. The fight-or-flight response and other automatic responses may become altered or muted, and coping hormones such as serotonin and other endorphins may become depleted, thus creating a decreased tolerance to pain.[4] If the fight-or-flight response persists in response to pain, the body can continue to release chemicals that cause muscle spasm and vessel constriction. This limits blood flow and oxygen delivery to the tissues where they are required for healing. This can perpetuate pain at the site. Further, the heart may continue to beat faster, and the person may respond with increased blood pressure. This can lead to an increased consumption of oxygen that would otherwise be used for normal, baseline bodily functions. The body needs to compensate. In an otherwise healthy person, this compensation may be noticeable as decreased energy or fatigue. A person who already has cardiovascular issues may not be able to compensate, and their health may become further compromised in response to persistent pain.

A persistent fight-or-flight response to acute pain may cause a person to develop and maintain a protective posture and to have shallow breathing. This is called splinting, an involuntary response in which a person tightens up to limit movement that causes pain.

Over time, the rib cage can develop limited movement, and the abdominal diaphragm, the muscle that needs to fully move up and down beneath the rib cage to generate airflow in the lungs, becomes tight and restricted. As a result, the person isn't getting oxygen deeply within their tissues when they take a breath. So there is a marginal deficit in oxygen delivery in the face of increased oxygen demand caused by pain. Another compensation occurs. The body runs on oxygen, and the body needs to compensate for decreased oxygen delivery with energy that would otherwise go toward normal biological functions. This might include corrective measures that would lead to the body normally healing the injury. In an otherwise healthy person, this compensation might be marginally noticeable as fatigue, but for a person who already has breathing difficulties due to asthma or COPD, this decreased capacity could lead to more respiratory episodes.

Normalizing the Pain Pathways

By now you may be wondering, *If I have chronic pain, how do I stop it and all the negative effects it is having on my body?* Again, you need to access and control the pain pathways in your body in as many strategic places as you can.

Frank Willard, professor of anatomy and neuroanatomy at the University of New England; John Jerome, a clinical pain psychologist at Michigan State University; and Mitchell Elkiss, a neurologist in southeast Michigan, suggest that the most complete approach to managing pain is a top-down and bottom-up process.[5] What this means is that if multiple points are switched on along a pain pathway going up to the brain, within the brain, and along the descending pathways to the body, then a person needs to address pain in both directions. This is critical in the diagnosis and treatment of chronic pain, and altering the ascending and descending pathways through medication, neuromodulation, manipulation, and retraining exercises are all strategies we will discuss.

Changing your brain and your response to pain are also key. The brain can modulate or affect pain by directing activity in the nerves and systems beneath it. While some changes within the pain pathway can be permanent, many changes can be reversed or corrected. If the nervous system can change for the negative, it can also change for the positive. This is good news.

So for effective treatment, it isn't usually just one pill, one injection, one routine, or one exercise that brings about change for healing. Effective treatment involves accessing as many points along the pain pathway as possible and normalizing the message. This is a multimodal approach and is what this book is about: implementing several simple but strategic changes in the way we think, what we expect, and what activities we engage in to respond to pain.

One of the greatest difficulties to overcome is a sense of a loss of control. But once you understand this process of addressing the pain message as it goes up to the brain and then down again, you will be more confident about ways to reduce pain. Research confirms that the more you feel you have control in your life, the more hope you have. Your pain experience can be explained, and you can better manage your pain.[6] The goal is to help you reestablish control in your battle against pain—one strategic step and one strategic change at a time.

5

The Five Most Common
Types of Pain

Acceptance doesn't mean resignation—it means understanding that something is what it is and that there's got to
be a way through it.

Michael J. Fox

In primary care medicine, much research has been done to better
understand what brings patients to the doctor. It can be an earache
or a common cold. Or it can be the need to address diabetes or to
control blood pressure. But the most common problem that brings
a patient to a physician is pain.

Headaches

Headaches are one of the most common pain complaints that
bring someone to see a physician or other health-care worker.
Narrowing down the cause of pain is often complex, requiring

thoughtful intervention. Perhaps more than any other pain condition, headaches can involve all types of pain—nociceptive, neuropathic, inflammatory, and psychogenic. Vascular components
can also be involved. Because of these complexities, treatment of
headaches usually requires a multimodal approach.

Tension headaches are the most common type of headaches.
Tension headaches are generally described as a tight band encir-
cling the head, causing a dull and aching head pain. Often, tenderness in the neck and upper shoulder muscles is also present. The
exact cause of tension headaches is uncertain.

Doctors used to think that tension headaches were due to stress
causing muscle contractions in the neck and head. However, research suggests that tension headaches are not necessarily the
result of distress or muscle contractions. More accurately, stress
and muscle tension over time can cause nerve fibers in the head
and neck to become more sensitized. As a result, there is a lowered
threshold for sending the nociceptive message and for feeling pain
in these areas. So while stress is considered chief among many
triggers for tension-type headaches, other triggers include fatigue,
overexertion, dehydration, alcohol, postural or muscle tension,
eye strain, sinus congestion, caffeine (excess or withdrawal), and
clenching teeth.

Cervicogenic headaches, or headaches caused by dysfunction
in the neck, have a different pain pattern than tension headaches.
These headaches usually occur on one side and are based on where
in the neck the dysfunction originates. They often occur after neck
trauma, such as after a car or whiplash-associated accident.

Cervicogenic headaches often contribute to or are found in
combination with other types of headaches. Cervicogenic headaches are usually persistent, steady pain as opposed to the throbbing pain that can occur with tension or migraine headaches.
They often are caused by certain movements of the neck, such
as turning the neck a certain way, coughing, sneezing, or taking
a deep breath. Cervicogenic headaches, in particular, respond

well to manipulation, physical therapy, and neck exercises, allowing for increased function, less pain, and less reliance on medication.[1]

Migraine headaches have many overlapping symptoms with tension-type and cervicogenic headaches, but while people often mistakenly brand a bad headache a migraine, they do have a pattern of their own and their underlying causes are quite different. Migraine headaches usually occur on one side, are throbbing, and can involve nausea, vomiting, and sensitivity to light and sound. They can last for hours, even days, and the pain can be severe, making it difficult to function in most daily activities.

Migraines may be preceded by a series of symptoms called a prodrome that often serves as a warning sign that a migraine is about to occur. These include constipation, yawning, increased thirst and urination, food cravings, and mood changes.[2] For some migraine sufferers, the prodrome is followed by an aura. The aura can involve visual changes such as bright areas in the visual field, flashes of light, shapes or a zigzag pattern, or even loss of the visual field. The aura can also involve neurologic signs such as jerking motions, a pins-and-needles sensation, difficulty speaking, and even weakness in the face or on one side of the body. After the migraine, there is also typically another prodrome period in which the person feels wiped out, depleted, and sometimes weak or confused.

Because migraines are caused by a different, more complex mechanism than are tension headaches and cervicogenic headaches, a completely different set of medication treatment strategies are needed, reinforcing the need to understand a person's type of pain in order to optimize treatment.

While headaches are painful, most are not life threatening. However, it is important to know when headaches can be dangerous. A headache that can be described as the worst pain in your life and had a sudden onset can be a hemorrhage, or bleeding within the brain, and is a medical emergency.

Headaches are also dangerous when they are associated with a fever and neck stiffness. In such cases, the cause might be a dangerous infection such as meningitis. Progressive or worsening neurologic changes such as difficulty expressing yourself, vocal hoarseness, difficulty swallowing, visual changes, and abnormal body sensation or weakness can suggest changes in the brain that could be related to cancer or other causes. That is why if you suffer from headaches, it is important to be evaluated by a physician in order to separate painful but benign headache symptoms from other symptoms that could indicate something more serious.

Another warning sign with headaches is when a stable headache pattern changes and the symptoms or locations of pain change. This could represent a different type of headache and perhaps a different cause that could be dangerous.

Low-back Pain

Low-back pain is another common musculoskeletal complaint that brings a person to see a physician or other health-care worker. While most back pain related to strain or overdoing eventually goes away as the body heals, back pain that persists is one of the most disabling pain conditions people experience.

Risk factors for low-back pain include being over forty, family history of back pain, previous back injury, lack of regular exercise, smoking, increased weight, postural strain, and emotional distress and psychological disorders. Occupational risk factors include long periods of sitting, lifting heavy objects, machine vibration, and twisting and bending. Interestingly, jobs that require a fair amount of standing and walking are less likely to cause low-back pain, probably because prolonged standing requires relative strength and stamina of core and postural muscles, and walking encourages blood and lymphatic flow and requires movement of the joints in the legs, pelvis, and vertebrae.

From a physician's standpoint, treating low-back pain can be difficult because the cause is often elusive and multifactorial. This is why it is important to determine the difference between pain caused by compression between vertebrae, inflammatory pain due to an injury or repetitive overuse, and neuropathic pain caused by tightness or injury around lumbar spinal nerve roots. Each can present differently, but more than one problem can also be present and contributing to the overall pain level.

Medication can be helpful when inflammation is involved or for muscle spasm in the short term, but often low-back pain isn't a medical problem per se. Research suggests that 97 percent of back pain has a mechanical cause, meaning that pain arises from stresses and strains on the back rather than from a disease.[3] Therefore, treatment plans including exercise and spinal manipulation are often useful, leading to less pain, less absence from work, reduced disability, less medication use, fewer physical therapy visits, and increased patient satisfaction.[4] (We will discuss manipulation further in chapter 11.) Sometimes, however, low-back pain is unresponsive to first-line treatments and requires procedural interventions. This is often the case with severe, persistent pain or when there is an increasing loss of strength or sensation.

It is important to be aware of what doctors refer to as "red flag" situations of back pain. These red flags include low-back pain in someone over the age of fifty; progressive loss of neurologic or musculoskeletal function; pain that awakens a person at night; pain in the presence of unexplained weight loss, night sweats, or fevers; and pain that doesn't lessen with rest. These symptoms could suggest nerve compression, cancer, or infections, so they need to be evaluated by your physician. Emergent situations can also occur with low-back pain. Low-back pain emergencies are associated with abrupt neurologic changes, changes in bowel or bladder function, including having accidents or an inability to urinate or defecate, and numbness in the saddle area of the groin and inner thigh. If you experience these symptoms in the context of your low-pack pain, you should seek medical attention right away.

Neck Pain

Neck pain is another common reason people see a physician. Since the neck is also part of the vertebral column, there is considerable overlap in how pain can develop compared to the low back. Like low-back pain, neck pain is usually caused by mechanical reasons such as compressive forces on vertebral joints, uneven muscle tension, and postural strain. Oftentimes, it is associated with muscle spasm in the neck or upper shoulder region. This type of neck pain, like low-back pain due to mechanical issues, also responds well to manipulation, stretching, and strengthening exercises. However, there are some key differences between low-back pain and neck pain.

First, low-back pain is more likely to resolve after strain because lumbar vertebrae are bigger and well-supported by surrounding structures. Neck strains tend to linger because the vertebral and supporting structures are not as strong and because the neck is responsible for supporting the weight of the head, thus making it more prone to injury with less force. When great forces are part of an injury, such as in a car accident, these tissues are much more vulnerable. Pain can therefore be caused from too much movement between vertebrae or instability in the injured tissue that supports the neck. This is why such care is taken to "clear" the neck after high-velocity accidents such as falls, car accidents, and other sorts of trauma.

Warning signs associated with neck pain are similar to those with low-back pain. They include numbness, tingling, weakness, and shooting pain, typically involving the arms but also potentially the legs. These are signs of cervical radiculopathy—pain, weakness, or numbness caused by compression or pinching of the nerve roots of the cervical spine that go to the upper extremities.

Other warning signs include neck pain associated with fever, severe muscle spasm, and masses as well as pain that is not alleviated by rest. These symptoms should be evaluated by your physician.

Osteoarthritis

Both neck and low-back pain can be caused by another common category of pain complaints: osteoarthritis. Osteoarthritis goes by several names. When involving the neck and low back, it is sometimes referred to as spondylosis. When it occurs in the knee, shoulder, or other joints, it is often referred to as degenerative joint disease. Perhaps the most descriptive name for all types is wear-and-tear arthritis.

Osteoarthritis is a progressive condition that involves loss of joint cartilage from decades of use or weight-bearing activities. It is the most common type of arthritis. Risk factors include older age, elevated weight, injury, and prolonged, abnormal movement of the joint structure. Oftentimes, inflammation can also be involved along the way to developing osteoarthritis and after it has settled in, but inflammation doesn't drive the degenerative process and people generally report stiffness more than swelling.

Over time, wear and tear can cause joints to become deformed. This deformity can cause not only loss of cartilage but also the development of abnormal bony formations at the joint called osteophytes. These limit the movement of the joint and can make the joint progressively stiff and painful. Most people with osteoarthritis experience stiffness and pain that are relieved with rest. However, in advanced stages of joint disease, the pain can become constant and severely limit daily activities and function.

It is important to know the difference between osteoarthritis and less common inflammatory disease conditions such as rheumatoid arthritis, systemic lupus erythematosus, and psoriatic arthritis of the musculoskeletal system. These are autoimmune diseases in which the inflammatory process is misdirected against normal tissue. The treatment approach medically can be vastly different, but addressing them from a behavioral, emotional standpoint can be similar to the approaches used with osteoarthritis or any other type of chronic pain.

Fibromyalgia

Fibromyalgia is different from other pain conditions in that it is categorized as a pain syndrome. There is not a specific, understood pathology or cause for why a person has pain. A person with fibromyalgia typically suffers from widespread, diffuse pain and tenderness, which are most commonly combined with fatigue and poor or disturbed sleep. Women develop fibromyalgia more often than men and generally report having tenderness to touch, pain with exertion, difficulties with hot or cold temperatures, and an increased pain response to painful stimulation that may not affect others as much. Other problems may also accompany fibromyalgia. Among them are headaches, irritable bowel symptoms, anxiety, depression, and cognitive impairment, sometimes referred to as "fibro fog."

Since there is no definable organic cause for fibromyalgia, the syndrome has been confounding doctors for decades. However, continuing research has increased our understanding of what within the body is causing pain. The developing consensus is that there is a central sensitization to pain. Research shows that people with fibromyalgia have altered pain modulation,[5] meaning there is an impaired ability to down-regulate the signals sent to and from the brain to reduce the sensation of pain. In addition, functional MRI studies show that the pain message is amplified where it is received in the brain and that fibromyalgia patients require less than half of the pressure stimulus to activate the pain sensation centers in the brain compared to the general public.[6]

How does all this happen? It is difficult to determine cause versus effect, but it is our sense, in working with people and piecing together research, that the sympathetic nervous system—the fight, flight, or freeze system—may be one of the primary contributors.

Research also shows that, compared to the general public, more people with fibromyalgia have suffered emotional trauma and physical or sexual abuse.[7] If someone suffers a highly stressful event or is persistently exposed to stressful situations, the fight, flight, or freeze mechanism may remain "switched on" at some level. The complex cross-wiring in the spinal cord between the fight, flight, or freeze nerve fibers, musculoskeletal nerve fibers, and sensory nerve fibers affects the muscles and fascia as well, which could lead to diffuse pain. Research also shows that there is an increase in and impaired regulation of cortisol, one of the primary stress hormones.[8] Cortisol levels could become dysregulated due to persistent stress.

For most of my (James's) fibromyalgia patients, this explanation resonates with them, but there isn't always abuse or emotional trauma in their backgrounds. Sometimes the stressful event was an injury, an accident, or an extended period taking care of a dying loved one. If you suffer from fibromyalgia, some of the tools in this book will be helpful for you. In order for your pain to get better, you may have to consider counseling and removing yourself from exposure to the stressful situation.

Red Flags for Pain

In describing the preceding conditions, we took care to describe when low-back pain, neck pain, and headaches indicate danger. While you should not try to diagnose yourself, we want to restate how important it is not to overlook serious symptoms of pain.

In general, any new, severe, or sudden pain in the chest, head, abdomen, or pelvis that creates fear or thoughts of impending doom should be evaluated immediately. Severe or unusual pain associated with a fever, chills, or night sweats is also a cause for evaluation. Further, any time you experience black or tar-like stools, blood in your stool, or vomiting that looks like coffee grounds, you must see a physician to evaluate for gastrointestinal bleeding, especially if you take nonsteroidal anti-inflammatory drugs (NSAIDs) for pain caused by inflammation.

Other symptoms may appear to be less urgent but still should be discussed with a physician. They include pain that is not alleviated with rest, pain that wakes you up at night or disrupts your sleep, and pain accompanied by unexplained weight loss. These could be signs of cancer-type pain. New pain that occurs over the age of fifty and new pain that occurs when you've had a history of cancer should also be evaluated.

Now that you have a foundational understanding of pain, you and your physician can fully discuss the types of pain you are experiencing, identify the patterns, and address your pain in the most appropriate and precise manner.

6

The Opioid Epidemic and Chronic Pain

The pain is there; when you close one door on it, it knocks to come in somewhere else.

Irvin D. Yalom

These days we hear a great deal about the opioid epidemic, the tens of thousands of overdose deaths, and the skyrocketing numbers of the addicted. It's not unreasonable to ask, How did we get to this point? Why have so many turned to opioids, considering how dangerous they can be? And, significantly, are opioids helpful when it comes to chronic pain?

What Are Opioids?

Opioids are a category of drugs that are derived naturally from the opium poppy plant. For most of civilization's written history, opium has been known to be effective in eliminating pain. It also induces a strong sense of euphoria. The parallel history of opium's use and abuse is as old as the substance itself.

Though opium's history spans thousands of years, one of its uses took a decidedly more narrowed, medicinal turn in the early 1800s when a German chemist named Friedrich Wilhelm Adam Sertürner isolated the active ingredient of the opium poppy plant and named it morphine, after Morpheus, the Greek god of dreams.

Morphine was used extensively as an analgesic (that is, causing an insensibility to pain without loss of consciousness). In America, it was used during the Civil War to treat soldiers who were gravely injured or mortally wounded in battle. However, in the decades that followed, it became clear that morphine was a powerful drug. Because of its potentially addictive properties, the federal government limited its use in one of the most far-reaching national legislations of its time, the Harrison Act of 1914.[1] This law limited the distribution of morphine and other opium derivatives by making them legally available only through physicians and pharmacists, who were required to be registered to prescribe.

The Harrison Act and various other regulations aimed at limiting opioid use set the tone in health care for most of the rest of the twentieth century. Physicians who prescribed opioid-derived pain medications such as morphine and oxycodone did so sparingly, in low doses, and for a short term to alleviate acute, demonstrable pain or to alleviate pain associated with terminal diseases such as cancer.[2]

A Miracle Becomes a Nightmare

Toward the end of the twentieth century, particularly in the 1990s, a few key dynamics came into play that changed the way physicians and other health-care providers prescribed opioid pain medication. The first was an industry-wide drive to improve best practices, particularly in how pain was treated. How a patient perceived the amount of pain they experienced was included as the "fifth vital sign." Though a subjective finding, it was documented alongside blood pressure, pulse, respiratory rate, and temperature at the top of a patient's chart.

During this same period, pharmaceutical companies introduced time-release opioid pain medications, which were marketed as safer than traditional opioids because of a more even dosing and controlled delivery of the medication within the body. Physicians and other health-care providers were told that these new medications had little to no addiction potential. There was essentially no ceiling on dose,[3] and the last twenty years saw a sharp increase in opioid prescribing.

This collective mind-set proved to be incorrect and led to what is now known as the opioid epidemic. For some people, addiction can occur with minimal exposure, and thus the original prescription can represent a gateway to addiction or illicit drug use.

Recent research suggests that some people may have a genetic predisposition to addiction to pain medication. In fact, it is estimated that 40 to 60 percent of the general population may be predisposed to addiction to opioid medication.[4] Some people process medication differently, causing an exaggerated response to the medication and a greater potential for intoxication.[5] Since this occurs within the reward areas of the brain, there is an instinctual drive to repeat the experience that outpaces rational thought. In the 1990s, when the expanded use of opioid medication occurred, more patients were exposed to opioids and at higher doses, affecting many of those predisposed to addiction.

In 2015, the amount of opioid pain medication prescribed was three times the amount prescribed in 1999.[6] During this same time period, there was also a precipitous rise in opioid-related deaths. The US Department of Health and Human Services reported the following data from 2017:

- 11.4 million people misused prescription opioids
- 2.1 million people had an opioid use disorder

- An estimated 130 people died *every day* from opioid-related overdoses
- 47,600 people died from opioid overdose
- 17,087 deaths were attributed to overdosing on common prescribed opioids
- 19,413 deaths were attributed to overdosing on synthetic opioids other than methadone
- 886,000 people used heroin
- 170,000 people used heroin for the first time
- 15,469 deaths were attributed to overdosing on heroin[7]

A renewed war on drugs has been driven by increased opioid addiction and greater numbers of those addicted seeking illicit drugs such as heroin. This has increased the demand, fueling an illegal drug trade. To be certain, other substances are also abused. Alcohol, for instance, claims more lives and consumes more health-care and societal resources than opioids. But because of the sharply rising trends related to prescription opioid use, there is more awareness of the opioid problem.

For people who depend on opioid pain medication to alleviate their pain, this current health crisis hits especially close to home. The majority of people who use prescribed opioid pain medication are not addicts. It is an unfortunate misperception held by some in the public, and even by some in the health-care industry, that the majority of opioid pain medication users are addicts. In fact, the opposite is true. Research indicates that most people who use prescription opioids for chronic pain use them appropriately—not to get high but for the appropriate pain-relieving effect.[8]

One of the discouraging consequences of the opioid epidemic is that people for whom these medications are appropriate and who could manage their use well face hurdles for pain relief in the form of increased doctors' visits, drug screens, pill counts, and other monitoring. Perhaps more discouraging is that the opioid crisis overshadows a much more vast epidemic of chronic pain.

Clearly, more has to be done, and more tools have to be implemented for us to get ahead of this problem as a society. Not only do we need to reconsider how opioid medication is prescribed but we also need to determine if other medical and nonmedical approaches might decrease opioid use.

It is important to understand when opioids are a good choice, when they are not, how to recognize if there is a problem with pain medication, and which treatment options are available if addiction has occurred.

How Opioids Work

To better understand how opioid medications work, think of them as keys floating in the bloodstream. When they attach to a receptor, they "unlock" the activity of that receptor. Opioid receptors reside throughout the body. At the spinal and peripheral nerve levels, opioids work to block the nociception message that would be sent to the brain that would translate into pain. When opioid pain medications interact with opioid receptors in the brain itself, they lock on and release neurotransmitters that diminish the perception of pain in the higher centers of the brain. In addition, reward centers are also stimulated, which creates sensations of pleasure.

Opioid pain medication can be a good choice for moderate to severe pain in acute or short-term circumstances, such as after trauma, surgery, or a bone fracture. In these cases, opioid medication should be used for as short a time as possible, perhaps just a few days. Opioids are also appropriate for treating pain associated with cancer. Sometimes when an injury occurs, though, using an anti-inflammatory medication is a better option because inflammation is likely what is causing the pain.

With chronic pain, opioids can sometimes be used to alleviate pain if they are managed carefully by a physician. The physician will ensure that the medication is appropriately covering the pain, isn't causing sedation, allows the patient to have increased functioning in their daily activities, and isn't causing an addiction. Opioids are not a good option when someone is having minimal amounts or no pain or if they are taking them because they are afraid of having pain. This practice can trigger the reward centers in the brain too strongly, causing a euphoric response that then becomes something the person will try to replicate, setting them up for addiction.

The Consequences of Overprescribing

One common example of misguided prescribing has been when a person has an outpatient procedure or an injury and a month's supply of opioids is prescribed. Overprescribing creates a greater opportunity for addiction in a patient who is susceptible to addiction. After the patient recovers from pain, they may have a large supply of opioids left in the medicine cabinet. What happens to that medication?

A recent study found that patients take only 28 percent of the opioid pills prescribed.[9] This has implications with regard to both teen utilization and giving medications to others. The National Survey on Drug Use and Health reported that 53 percent of the time opioid pain medication that is used by a person for nonmedical purposes is obtained free from a friend, and 84 percent of the time, the prescription for the medication that becomes diverted is from a single doctor.[10]

Whether treating pain with medication, an injection, or manual manipulation, you and your physician need to have the same goals. Recall that the main goal isn't always to be pain-free but to increase function. This guideline is especially important when dealing with opioid medication.

Pharmacologically speaking, it is generally possible to give enough opioid pain medication to completely eliminate pain. The problem is that when the goal is to have no pain, oftentimes the amount of medication required to reach that goal either has too many side effects or is otherwise harmful. Over time, too much medication creates a severe decline in functional capacity, and the risk for addiction increases.

To increase function, there must, of course, be less pain. But you must also shift your focus away from the pain and toward the things you can do. The more your attention is diverted from the pain, the less pain you will feel. When you function better, you feel more capable in life. This is both encouraging and empowering and helps restore a sense of control that was lost to pain.

By maintaining or increasing your activities of daily life, you preserve motion in your body—your back, your knees, your neck— that would otherwise be lost. A colleague of ours has an adage: "Motion is life." When we move less to protect a painful area, we lose motion not only in the protected area but also in almost every other area as well. As a result, the pain actually increases or pain develops in other areas. We will discuss this more in chapter 11. The point here is that you and the physician prescribing pain medication must be vigilant to create clear and reasonable goals to decrease pain and increase function, while at the same time, minimizing side effects or the potential for addiction.

Aspects of Addiction

Recent research suggests that some people may have a genetic predisposition to addiction to pain medication. As stated, it is estimated that 40 to 60 percent of the general population may be predisposed to addiction to opioid medication because their bodies process medication differently, causing them to have an exaggerated response to the medication.[11]

Because of the inherent risks associated with opioid medication use, it is important to understand certain terms. Opioid tolerance occurs when a person uses opioid medication on a chronic basis and an increased dose is required to achieve the same pain-relieving effect. Over time, a slow loss of active receptor sites for opioid medication occurs as a result of repeated exposure. In addition, there is a decrease in the affinity of the remaining opioid receptors. As a result, more medication is needed to have the same effect with pain, and the amount can continue to edge upward. A person who has a physical dependence on opioid medication will demonstrate withdrawal symptoms if the medication is discontinued abruptly. However, this is a normal physiologic response to the absence of a medication to which the body has become accustomed and should not, by itself, be considered a sign of substance abuse or addiction.[12]

According to the National Institutes of Health, opioid addiction is a chronic brain disease that causes a person to compulsively seek out drugs, even though the medication causes self-harm and the person experiences ongoing negative consequences.[13] Substance abuse is a broader term and includes but is not specific to opioid medication. It is the inappropriate use of an illegal substance or the use of a legal substance excessively or for purposes other than that for which it was prescribed.

It is important to understand that tolerance, physical dependence, and withdrawal symptoms can all occur in a person who is using opioid medication as prescribed and in an appropriate manner in order to manage pain. It is equally important to recognize when a person may not be using medication properly or has lost control.

The fifth edition of the *Diagnostic and Statistical Manual of Mental Disorders* defines opioid use disorder as "a problematic pattern of opioid use leading to clinically significant impairment or distress as manifested by at least two of the following, occurring within a 12-month period:

1. Opioids are often taken in large amounts or over a longer period of time than intended.
2. There is a persistent desire or unsuccessful effort to cut down or control opioid use.

3. A great deal of time is spent in activities necessary to obtain the opioid, use the opioid, or recover from its effects.

4. Craving, or a strong desire or urge to use opioids.

5. Recurrent opioid use results in failure to fulfill major role obligations at work, school, or home.

6. Continued opioid use despite having persistent or recurrent social or interpersonal problems caused or exacerbated by the effects of opioids.

7. Important social, occupational, or recreational activities are given up or reduced because of opioid use.

8. Recurrent opioid use in situations in which it is physically hazardous.

9. Continued opioid use despite knowledge of having a persistent or recurrent physical or psychological problem that is likely to have been caused or exacerbated by the substance.

10. Tolerance, as defined by either of the following:

    a. A need for markedly increased amounts of opioids to achieve intoxication or desired effect.

    b. A markedly diminished effect with continued use of the same amount of an opioid.

11. Withdrawal, as manifested by either of the following:

    a. The characteristic opioid withdrawal syndrome.

    b. Opioids (or a closely related substance) are taken to relieve or avoid withdrawal symptoms."[14]

What Drives Addiction Behavior?

One of the most commonly held misperceptions that occurs with any addiction is the thought, *I could quit at any time*. While this may be true at the beginning of treatment with opioids, it changes as use becomes more chronic. The decisional part of the brain is still working well before use becomes compulsive. However, once compulsive use begins, neuropathways are changed in the brain. The need for reward becomes stronger, and decision-making becomes less effective. This is when family members, friends, and others begin to notice drug-seeking behaviors, loss of control, and panic about not having the medication.

One of the common experiences those who become addicted to opioid medication have is that the absence of the medication makes them desperate to have more. If someone's body is used to certain levels of opioid medication and then goes without it, the withdrawal symptoms are severely pronounced. One person described withdrawal as having the flu but multiplying that experience by one thousand. Part of the desperate behavior that leads to and is associated with addiction is not related to the euphoria that opioid medication can bring. It is because the person will do anything, even something illegal, such as seek illicit drugs like heroin, to avoid the suffering associated with withdrawal.

When people become addicted, functional MRIs can show what happens inside the brain. In addicts, this test shows more baseline activity in the basal ganglia region of the brain and reduced baseline activity in the anterior cingulate gyrus portion of the prefrontal cortex. This has profound significance in explaining the compulsive and impulsive behaviors that are associated with addiction.

The basal ganglia region, where opioids act and where dopamine is released, is where the reward centers of the brain reside. This area is driven more by instinct and pleasure than by rational thought. Conversely, the area that shows less activity, the prefrontal cortex, is where discernment, rational thought, and decision-making with regard to reward and punishment occur. This information is critical to understanding what is occurring in the mind of someone who is addicted to pain medication or most any type of opioid drug. Those who are addicted are biochemically driven more by instinct, reward, and avoidance of suffering than by reason and accountability.[15] This means that addiction and addiction behavior are not moral failures. Addiction and addiction behavior cannot be overcome simply by exercising enough willpower. The decisions that addicts make are survival driven. They are driven both by avoidance of suffering and by the reward of the drug.

The Use of Medically Assisted Treatment

All is not lost. One of the approaches that can help people get off opioid medications—medication assisted treatment (MAT)—involves using medication combined with a wide range of services, including counseling and behavioral therapy, to provide a comprehensive approach to substance abuse. MAT is used to treat opioid use disorder, including heroin and prescription pain medication addiction. The opioid treatment programs (OTPs) are broader programs that are not necessarily medical but accredited by the Substance Abuse and Mental Health Services Administration (SAMHSA) "to prevent, reduce, or eliminate the use of controlled or illegal substances, the potential criminal activity related to their use, and/or spread of infectious disease."[16]

Health providers who participate in OTPs must undergo stringent training in order to receive certification to provide care, primarily because opioid medications, specifically methadone and buprenorphine, are used as part of the treatment program. These medications have been shown to dramatically decrease the urge to use opioids and thus provide people who suffer from opioid use disorder a chance to recover from the disease of addiction.

Methadone is a synthetic opioid that can be used for pain but has a slightly different mechanism and receptor profile than other opioids. As a result, it changes how the brain and nervous system respond to pain. It is helpful in treatment programs because it reduces the symptoms of opioid withdrawal and blocks the euphoric effects, suppressing and reducing the craving for these drugs. While withdrawal from opioids is rarely fatal, it can be severely uncomfortable or even painful to endure. Methadone works well because it allows a person to decrease or eliminate the use of and to detoxify from illicit or addictive opioid medication without the need for hospitalization. When prescribed and taken appropriately, methadone also has no adverse effect on a patient's cognitive function, physical capability, or ability to work. The downside of methadone is that it must be dispensed and supervised in a highly structured clinic. This limits convenience and access.

The other primary OTP medication used to help people reduce or eliminate the use of opioids is buprenorphine—a mixed type of opioid medication that has a slightly different mode of action compared to heroin and other prescription opioid medications. It binds strongly to opioid receptor sites but causes a significantly less euphoric response. If a person uses buprenorphine, other opioids can't bind to the receptor site. In this way, buprenorphine suppresses and reduces the craving for other opioids. A benefit of buprenorphine is that it does not have to be prescribed or monitored in a specific facility such as a methadone clinic. Rather, a physician who is trained and credentialed can prescribe and monitor buprenorphine from their office. This greatly increases access for treatment for those who are struggling with opioid addiction.

Finally, naloxone is often prescribed for those who suffer major addiction behaviors and for whom overdose is a serious concern. This medication is used primarily as a rescue medication that family members, friends, or loved ones can administer by injection or intranasally if an active overdose has occurred. The medication quickly restores normal breathing to someone whose breathing has slowed or stopped. It can save a life.

The opioid epidemic is a battle yet to be won. An interprofessional and multifaceted approach is needed. If addiction becomes a problem when dealing with chronic pain, it must be addressed and most likely will require professional help.

7

Not All in Your Head—Or Is It?

> The merest schoolgirl, when she falls in love, has Shakespeare or Keats to speak her mind for her; but let a sufferer try to describe a pain in his head to a doctor and language at once runs dry.
>
> Virginia Woolf

One of the most famous and recognized paintings in the world is permanently displayed at the Museum of Modern Art in New York City. It is Vincent van Gogh's *The Starry Night*. Every day hundreds of people pass by the wall that holds this exquisite work of art. Everyone who stops and looks sees the exact same painting. Yet the experience of the art differs from person to person.

When I (Linda) look at that painting, I see chaos and depression in the swirling orbs. A physicist may look and marvel at the swirling clouds, seeing in the painting a mathematical theory of turbulence. Some people may be moved by the painting's beauty, cry, and become highly emotional. Others may notice the overwhelming night sky and feel afraid. Perhaps some people focus on the eleven yellow orbs that illuminate the sky. Others may focus on the illusion of constant motion. Regardless of the interpretation, the stimulus of the painting is the same for all the people who see it. It is a physical masterpiece of art, but reactions to it are varied and subjective.

Pain is like a painting. The pain stimulus may be the same for people—a broken leg, a bee sting, a twisted arm, back pain, a headache, and so on—but the reaction to the pain stimulus can vary from person to person. This is because the reaction is influenced by many factors. While pain, like the painting, is very real, the *perception* of pain is subjective and unique. Pain cannot be quantified objectively because it involves feelings, behaviors, thoughts, memories, and personal experiences, all resulting in a unique, subjective response to pain.

Pain Is in the Brain, but Not the Way You Think

If you are pain-free at the moment, try to reproduce a time of great pain. If you have ever given birth, that pain is an easy one to use as an example. Can you feel the pain? Can you bring the actual pain back to memory? You can remember the pain stimulus (that is, the birth experience) and all the emotions and thoughts around the experience that lead to the memory, but you cannot reproduce the actual experience. You remember childbirth as being incredibly painful, but it is a memory, not an immediate pain experience. Thank goodness—or most of us would opt to have this experience only once in our lives! The fact that people give birth more than once has to do with our inability to re-create the actual pain experience. The brain remembers that experience as painful, but it cannot reproduce the physical experience of pain in the here and now. However, the brain does store emotions, thoughts, and beliefs around a pain experience and develops a pain perception related to that experience.

Recall that your brain is part of a body protection system that is ready to sound the pain alarm if it detects threat. A good system will activate when it detects a threat or danger and will turn off once the threat has passed. In addition, your brain learns from negative experiences and remembers them in order to avoid future pain.

When there is a threat to your body, the threat itself does not generate pain. Pain is a result of the *perception* that comes from the activity of the brain. Here is how this works. When there is an injury or tissue threat, the spinal cord sends the signal to the brain stem and activates other reflexes in the autonomic nervous system and the endocrine system of your body. Still, this doesn't mean you experience pain. It is when the spinal cord sends the signal to the traffic controller of the brain, the thalamus, that pain becomes a reality. A number of regions of the brain are activated, and pain is felt. Pain is in the brain and remembered. The feeling of pain involves past learning experiences and the current emotions you feel. Because of your unique experiences and the emotions you feel, pain is different from person to person and can change over time.

The takeaway here is that pain can be good and protective, but at other times, it can be chronic and a signal that something is wrong in the way pain is being processed. Constant alarms going off due to chronic inflammation or the neural highways of the spinal cord and brain changing and becoming more sensitive are signals that something's wrong. The protective system is turned on, thinking there is a threat. That protective system includes sensory, emotional, cognitive, and body sensation processing. The neural circuits are changed. They have rewired and continue to fire. Your state of mind is altered and influencing the way you perceive your body.

Retraining the Brain

To better understand this, let's say you experience a painful event like falling off a bicycle. The memory of that is stored in multiple connections in your brain. It stays there if revisited now and then or if you reflect on the experience.

Then every time you think about falling off your bike and re-member the pain, the memory becomes stronger and more vivid. This is a process called reconsolidation. Eventually, just the thought of the bike can trigger pain. But every time you recall the memory, your mind has the ability to hack that memory and alter or reset it. So, for example, if the next time you saw the bike you stayed calm when remembering the pain situation, this new calm response blocks the neurotransmitter norepinephrine and stops the fight-or-flight (alarm) response. Now you have dampened that memory and prevented it from being associated with negative emotions. This is important because negative emotions associated with pain ramp it up. If you change your emotions and thoughts, you can reset the pain memory in a new way and lessen the pain. This is one reason mind-body treatments work. You can rewrite your pain story and dampen the pain.

Chronic pain activates parts of the brain related to memory and emotion. Again, think of the brain as having a system of highways. Chronic pain drives on some of those highways over and over again. The highways that get used the most become the most efficient, and they become part of your memory and emotions just like a familiar route to the grocery store. To rid yourself of chronic pain, you have to exit certain highways and drive on new ones.

To change directions, consider your thoughts. Thoughts are powerful and travel through your brain in specific ways and can change your brain. If you change the way you think, you can change how you feel pain. It has been said that if you change your thoughts, you can change your world. This is an important idea in dealing with chronic pain. Attending to your thoughts and making them positive can calm your nervous system and cultivate patterns of thought that turn down the volume on pain. It is a matter of learn-ing to train your brain.

The brain is complex and tricky, though. It has a hard time forgetting pain. Pain memories leave their mark on the nervous system and lead to hypersensitivity to more pain or even touch related to those memories. But we just learned that a memory can be modified and a new version saved on the hard drive of the mind. Pain is like a text document in the brain. You can revise your pain document and hit Save. Then it has been altered and changed. When you approach pain in new ways, you can teach your brain to rewire away from chronic pain. The strategies to do this are presented in later chapters.

When it comes to chronic pain, multiple factors are involved. Typically, there isn't a single cause or cure. Pain is not a good indicator of what is actually going on in the body because it is a perception capable of being modified in good or not so good ways. Neuroscientist V. S. Ramachandran goes so far as to say that, metaphorically, pain is a body's opinion. And it is an opinion we listen to because it speaks loudly at times. It makes up its mind and then sends messages to the brain that impact the sensitivity and behavior of the nerves.[1]

Pain messages travel up and down your central nervous system. Your nerves send pain messages, but your brain is able to tell your nerves how much of the signal to send up and then amplify it or calm it down. The brain is in charge and tells you what to feel.

Pain serves a function, but it can be overprotective. Thus, part of the problem is that the danger associated with pain is real, but it may be an exaggeration because of the faulty signaling occurring. This is why finding a new social context for the pain, lessening anxiety, or engaging in deep breathing can help change the pain perception. These types of changes help us cope and direct our experiences in different ways. Convince your brain that you are coping and safe, and your pain calms down. On the other hand, if your brain believes there is a threat, you are going to hurt. That's how the brain works.

Along with the physical sensation of pain, you also have emotional reactions to pain that you might not be aware of. Those emotional reactions also influence pain perception. Emotional feelings can determine what you feel in your body. The more positive and optimistic you are, the better you will feel and will cope with chronic pain. However, negative emotions can feed the cycle of pain. Then, chronic pain feeds negative emotions. It all becomes a vicious cycle.

But you aren't powerless. You can reprogram the neural pathways in your brain by using your mind. Your mind controls the mental processes that create thoughts, feelings, beliefs, perceptions, and attitudes. Your mind can change the way the brain functions. You can make up your mind to think, behave, and feel certain things in order to reduce the threat of stress, anxiety, and fear. Again, that doesn't mean your pain is just psychological. Rather, that your mind can play a role in your perception of pain.

To better understand this process, think of your brain as a very busy city with many superhighways. One highway signals physical pain. Another signals pain perception. According to a study at the University of Colorado at Boulder,[2] you can use your thoughts to help modulate pain because thoughts travel on a separate brain highway from the highway that signals physical pain. This means that two different highways in the brain contribute to pain perception. One highway sends signals regarding the intensity of painful stimuli to regions of the brain associated with pain perception. The other highway, which involves brain regions related to emotions and motivation, can be used to cognitively regulate pain perception. As a result, you can use your mind to alter and manage your pain perceptions. Since the perception of pain is in your brain (a product of your nervous system), your brain determines pain.

Part of the work in dealing with chronic pain is desensitizing your brain so you can turn down the volume on pain. When you address the factors that influence the experience of pain—like emotions and thoughts—you can often reverse how the nervous system is sensitized.

Can I Think Away My Pain?

The brain uses information from the senses, such as vision and touch, to modulate pain. Learning how to help your brain and change your perception of pain is essential to dealing with chronic pain. Since chronic pain involves neurological changes, work is needed to deal with those changes. We are not suggesting that you can just think away your pain, because chronic pain is more than thoughts. However, your thoughts, feelings, and behaviors can help moderate your pain and change your pain perception.

As we will discuss later, the more you focus on your pain, the worse you will feel. Muscle tension and stress contribute to feeling out of control and make pain worse. Negative feelings begin to cascade, resulting in depression and coping problems. The brain and the body are stressed and stuck in the "pain on" mode. Fear memories are laid down in the brain and available to be retrieved later. The long-term experience of pain gets implanted in your memory. With persistent pain, your spinal cord amplifies pain and your brain reorganizes. This is how your pain perception develops. Then you learn to anticipate painful events, maybe to minimize or avoid them.

Now please understand that reacting to pain isn't abnormal or a pathological process. Your feelings are real. The rewiring of your brain is telling your body an unpleasant pain story.

Most people are unaware of how or when chronic pain becomes a reality. Usually there is a triggering event such as tissue damage or nerve pain. When the body is confronted with stress, it tries to adapt to that stress. The brain reacts and tries to manage the experience. As a result, chemical and structural brain changes occur.

With chronic pain, the brain is strained and alters such things as perception, emotion, cognition, learning, and motivation, which are also tied to other body functions such as sleep. When we feel the strain, we want to avoid and protect ourselves. Pain is recorded as traumatic, and the nervous system automatically responds. Now the initial triggering event has progressed to a chronic pain state, altering the way we think, feel, and behave.

You lose energy and your capacity to cope when dealing with chronic pain. You become more sensitive to what is happening in your body and more aware of the pain. This heightened pain sensitivity decreases pain tolerance.[3] A type of fear learning begins that we will discuss in chapter 14. You seek relief but don't get it—and this leads to more stress. This felt loss of control is telling your body that it can't adapt to all the stress. It is too much. Chronic stress then makes you feel worse. This emotional stress is learned and remembered.

While you can't simply think away your pain, you can influence it tremendously when you better understand it. You can alter your pain perception—with changes in multiple areas of your life—and begin to undo the effects of chronic pain.

So let's find ways to help your nervous system and make a painful area feel better. Be confident that you can influence your perception of pain. This will include an assessment of your beliefs, thoughts, emotions, and behaviors. Your mental state can be extremely helpful in reducing pain. There are things you can do to reinterpret your experiences of pain. You can rewire your brain and eliminate or weaken learned pathways through nonpharmacological treatments.

8

Stress and Pain

Things hurt more when you're stressed or sad, and the increased pain makes you both stressed and sad. The way out of this vicious circle is a wholesale change to how you perceive fear, suffering and setbacks.

Rob Heaton

"I'm stressed out, tired, exhausted." These words reflect a growing state of stressed-out lives, and people in all walks of life are affected. If you feel overwhelmed by the demands of family and work, you are not alone.

Stress is a by-product of our postmodern life. We feel we have too little time, too few resources, and a lack of control over most things in our lives. Stress can be related to life transitions, the environment, individual growth, a desire for healing, or a perception of things. Stress can be generated by an event such as a death, an illness, or a bad decision. Some stressful events, like the birth of a baby, are positive and predictable. Others, such as a natural disaster and an injury, are not. When stress is negative and unpredictable, it can be harder to manage.

How we react to stress is the key to keeping it in check. If we carry stress in our bodies and minds, it disrupts our sense of well-being—and interferes with the mental and physical rest we need. Unmanaged stress can lead to the development of anxiety disorders, depression, and physical symptoms, including pain.

Stress is a part of life and can be a good motivator, but too much of it or ongoing stress can be problematic. When stress is present, the brain releases chemicals and hormones; heart rate and blood pressure increase; the immune system is activated; the throat becomes dry and tense; the skin becomes cool, clammy, or sweaty; and the digestive system shuts down. Your neck, back, shoulders, and head can hurt. You become tense and constricted in your muscles, which leads you to feel tired. Chronic stress causes repeated surges of cortisol, resulting in cortisol dysfunction and inflammation.[1] Muscles tense up, making the pain worse. Your brain has trouble filtering your pain signals. Over time, your stressed brain gets more and more sensitized to processing pain and it takes less and less stimuli to experience it.[2] The body wants balance. Pain and stress disrupt this. The body attempts to adapt to stress and pain, but after awhile, it is challenged by both. Pain and stress create constant wear and tear on the body and emotions.

The body is designed to fight unpleasant sensations related to pain. As a simplified example, suppose you have back pain and the stress of it causes muscle tension. This can produce pressure on nerves in the area. The pressure leads to more tension and stress and increases pain even more. You are in a vicious cycle of pain and stress. Then you feel irritable and anxious, which turns up the volume on pain even more. Ultimately, chronic stress makes you more vulnerable to pain and makes pain worse.[3]

The Brain's Role

The brain plays a role in the processing of stress and chronic pain. When our body determines a situation is stressful, it activates the part of our autonomic nervous system that goes into a fight-or-flight response. This triggers the activation of our central stress reponse system called the hypothalamic-pituitary-adrenal (HPA) axis and leads to a release of adrenal glucocorticoids.[4] These hormones have receptors in the emotional processing centers of the brain called the limbic brain and impact cell functioning.[5] Perceived stress causes the limbic brain to remember and pay attention and to decide to flee or stay in a situation. All of this works together to protect you from danger and to help you learn what is not safe. Basically, chronic stress causes your nervous system to go into survival mode and have difficulty returning to a calmer state.

Researchers at the University of Montreal studied the relationship between stress and pain from a neurobiological standpoint. They conducted a pain study and found a relationship between the size of the structure in the brain called the hippocampus and a vulnerability to stress. The smaller the volume of the hippocampus (the center of memory and spatial navigation), the more stress (higher cortisol levels) and, consequently, the more pain.[6] And there was more activity in the part of the brain (anterior parahippocampal gyrus) related to anxiety over anticipation of pain.

Why Some People Are Less Resilient with Regard to Stress and Pain

Over the years, we have observed that some people are more resilient than others when it comes to stress and pain. Others seem to go into a downward spiral more quickly. Here are a few of the reasons for these differences.

Because the mind and the body are so connected, a history of physical and psychological trauma puts a person more at risk for chronic pain.[7] Sexual abuse is especially difficult and can predispose a person to chronic pain. A history of childhood adversity, including such things as divorce, family conflict, abuse, and so on, can also trigger or make pain worse.[8] The same is true with adult conflict and victimization. These are examples of chronic stress, which are associated with negative memories that are tough to extinguish. Thus, trauma can raise anxiety and be a route to chronic pain.

Post-traumatic stress disorder (PTSD) is also seen more often in people with chronic pain.[9] Negative emotions associated with PTSD are one factor that can intensify pain. But another reason for this increase in pain can be because the pain itself is a continual reminder or a trigger event for the trauma once experienced. This then makes the PTSD worse and can result in the person reducing physical activity, leading to possible physical disability. This is because trauma and chronic pain share a common denominator—the nervous system. Both make the nervous system more reactive. When the nervous system is more sensitized, the person is at a greater risk for chronic pain. Cognitive behavioral therapy (CBT) can help manage chronic pain when PTSD or other types of trauma have been experienced.[10] We will come back to this in chapter 19.

A Positive Response to Stress

One solution to overcoming chronic stress is eliminating stress where and when you can. For example, could you say no to one more activity in your life that might bring undue stress? Could you work on a troubled marriage? Could you stop putting yourself into debt? Sometimes the best stress management technique is eliminating certain stressors in your life.

Other times you cannot get rid of the source of stress and have to cope with whatever happens. When stress can't be eliminated, consider your resources. Resources are those things that can help you cope with stress when it hits. They include your family, friends, spouse and community, finances, status, power, patience, faith, and so on.

Reducing life stress will improve the quality of your life. Why? Physically, stress drains you. Psychologically, stress affects your ability to think clearly, remember things, make good decisions, and regulate your emotions. Most importantly, eliminating stress can physically alter your vulnerability to recurring pain.

There is overlap between your neuroanatomy and your physiology when it comes to chronic pain and chronic stress.[11] Prolonged stress can intensify your body's reaction to stress. You become hypervigilant to stress and activate the HPA axis. Inflammation then facilitates yet more pain.[12]

Stress of all types can make pain worse if it's not managed or controlled. A key component of living beyond pain is to manage stress and develop good coping skills. We are capable of modifying what we perceive as stressful and of responding to stress in adaptive ways. Also, the more you can eliminate or avoid stress triggers, the better your stress management will be. Stress affects your pain and dials it up if not well managed. Because stress management is so important, we have devoted an entire chapter to help you minimize, manage, and eliminate stress (see chapter 16).

9

The Importance of Marginal Gains

When we finally reached out for help, we then started to make progress through a series of baby steps that put us back on a path of hope, health, and happiness.

Dr. Gregory Jantz

The American Chronic Pain Association has a great visual when it comes to thinking about pain. When you have pain, you are like a car with four flat tires. When medical treatment is used alone, it is like inflating one of the tires. But all four tires need to be inflated so that the car can run smoothly. Much can be done to get the car moving again—to help you manage pain and lead a productive, satisfying, and happy life. A combination of therapies and interventions is usually needed. Once the tires are filled and the car is moving again, it needs to keep moving down the road of life.[1]

While all of us would probably opt to eliminate chronic pain, the complete absence of pain is not necessarily a realistic goal. In fact, we are not promised a pain-free life. A more attainable goal is to reduce pain and learn to manage it in a way that allows you to do more of what you want and need to do. Ultimately, you want to increase your functioning, improve the quality of your life, and reduce your sense of suffering.

Now that you better understand the science of chronic pain, you know that you should not blame yourself for your pain. Your body has been changed and needs help to both modulate and change your pain. This seems like a large task, but the truth is that several strategic, even small changes can make a big difference in getting ahead of your pain. The way to do this is beautifully illustrated by a strategy from the world of cycling.

In cycling, the Tour de France is considered the premier annual event. This grueling, twenty-one-stage contest lasts over three weeks as cyclists from around the globe race through French villages and historic cities, the countryside, and even the mountain ranges of the Alps and the Pyrenees.

This is not just a competition between riders but also a competition to overcome the elements of heat, rain, dehydration, and fatigue—and somehow avoid a high-speed collision. The race has been likened to running a marathon every day. Simply participating in the race is considered a national honor in the competing countries. Winning it bestows legendary status. When the cyclists cross the line on day twenty-three in Paris, they typically will have logged over twenty-two hundred miles.

Winners have come from many countries—France, Belgium, and Spain have won the most[2]—but for the first one hundred years of the event, no one from Great Britain had ever won. That all changed in 2009.

After a century of British futility with the Tour de France, a British telecommunications company assembled Team Sky in 2009, Great Britain's first professional road-racing team. Partnering with Dave Brailsford, who was the performance director for the Olympic gold medal–winning British cycling track teams, Team Sky was established with the ambitious goal of winning the Tour within five years.

What Brailsford—who earned undergraduate degrees in sports science and psychology and a master's in business administration—brought to Team Sky was a concept borrowed from the business world: the concept of marginal gains. Brailsford explained, "The whole principle came from the idea that if you broke down everything you could think of that goes into riding a bike, then improved it 1 percent, you will get a significant improvement when you put them all together."[3]

Based on this concept of marginal gains, Brailsford and his team looked at everything in the cycling process. Not only did they look at which were the best bikes, tires, cranks, and pedals but they also evaluated rider aerodynamics in a wind tunnel. They looked at where the team stayed overnight while on tour and what pillows worked best to help provide a good night's rest. Brailsford's team researched best practices to avoid illness and fatigue, including meals and in-race nutrition and hydration, race-day recovery strategies, and the way cyclists routinely washed their hands. They even painted the inside of their gear trailer white so that they would be able to notice and minimize the accumulation of dirt and debris so that the cycling equipment would function optimally. Every part of the process of the Tour and cycling was evaluated. No stone was left unturned.

The cumulative results of improving every last detail, even just a little bit, were staggering. It didn't take the British team five years to win the Tour de France; it took them three. In 2012, Bradley Wiggins and Team Sky brought the first Tour victory home to England. Fellow Briton Chris Froome led Team Sky to victory in 2013, 2015, 2016, and 2017, while teammate Geraint Thomas won in 2018. Team Sky has won the Tour de France an unprecedented six times in seven years. Other teams have taken notice and are following suit in their process to change and improve.

How does all of this exciting cycling news apply to you? The process of marginal gains can be applied to pain control too. When several small changes are made in a person's life and consistently applied, even changes that require very little effort, the aggregate difference over time can be life changing. Marginal gains win the game of life. They are doable and put you in a race you can win over time.

There are a couple more things we can learn from Team Sky. When Chris Froome won the Tour de France in 2017, he did so without winning any of the twenty-one stages of the race.[4] This proved to be a good strategy. By viewing it as a twenty-three-day race, Froome and his team were steady, strategic, and focused over the entirety of the event instead of going full gas on any one stage. A similar approach needs to be taken when applying the concept of marginal gains to your pain. In this book, there are many strategies that will help you reduce your pain. But don't overdo and then fade out. Start with a few ideas that resonate with you—even ones that may be easy to do—and then be disciplined in sticking with them. Then once you've achieved a marginal gain and have begun to see benefits, add another, then another, and so on. This will give you momentum and success you can build on for the long haul.

The second point here is that it *is* a long haul. It may take a while for you to see change, but hopefully the way things are today will be a little bit different tomorrow. The way things are tomorrow will be different a month from now. And the way things are a month from now will look vastly different in a year. Keep your best vision of your life in front of you, make incremental changes, don't give up, and you can see big changes over time.

We are providing you with the factors that surround pain, from the intricate and complex neuropathways that convey the message of pain; to how your body, mind, and emotions respond to injury and distress; to the daily habits that contribute to pain relief. The next section of the book focuses on multiple ways to become like those cyclists and work on marginal gains. Small changes in strategic places can increase your capacity for a healthier, more functional life and give you hope to live beyond pain.

PART 2

TOOLS *for* PAIN MANAGEMENT

10

Traditional Approaches to Pain Management

If opening your eyes, or getting out of bed, or holding a spoon, or combing your hair is the daunting Mount Everest you climb today, that is okay.

Carmen Ambrosio

There is no one single approach that effectively takes care of pain. True relief is not a simple matter of finding the right pill. Instead, you may need various approaches to manage your pain.

This chapter describes traditional approaches to pain management. In general, traditional approaches can be divided into three areas: medical management, noninvasive modalities, and invasive procedures. Choosing the appropriate approach depends on what level of pain you are experiencing, what has been tried before, what has worked, and what hasn't. Treatment also needs to be highly personalized and based on a clear understanding of the root cause of your pain and other factors that may be contributing to it. Working with your doctor to address the cause is important so your treatment doesn't become an exercise in symptom management but focuses on increased function and quality of life.

Medical Management

Medical management refers to controlling pain through the use of drugs. These include both over-the-counter and prescribed medications that are generally taken by mouth.

Over-the-Counter (OTC) Drugs

Pain relievers that are available over-the-counter (OTC) are typically used intermittently for short-term relief of mild to moderate pain conditions such as headaches, low-back pain, and arthritis. Pain relievers generally act by decreasing the perception of pain in the brain or in the messaging network in the nervous system or by blocking the production of specific chemicals that may cause pain within the body.

Acetaminophen is the most commonly used pain reliever, but it also functions as a fever reducer. Interestingly, the exact mechanism of how it works in the body is not known, but it is thought to inhibit enzymes that lead to the production of inflammation.[1]

Acetaminophen is generally well tolerated and effective in treating pain, but care must be used not to exceed the daily dose limit on the bottle (3,000 mg per day). Overdosage can cause liver toxicity, which can be fatal. While following the dose limit on the bottle should keep you safe, one hidden danger is that acetaminophen is an active ingredient in more than six hundred OTC and prescription medications. So it is important to read the ingredients list on medications to ensure that you are not doubling up.

Anti-inflammatories are a second type of OTC medication. Inflammation, as discussed earlier, is part of the body's normal, protective response to injury, infection, or other harmful stimuli. Aspirin, ibuprofen, and naproxen are common examples of nonsteroidal anti-inflammatory drugs (NSAIDs) that work by blocking certain chemicals produced in the body that cause inflammation. NSAIDs are effective in treating classic arthritis pain caused by joint overuse or long-term wear and tear. They are also useful in treating acute pain from minor injuries, such as a sprained ankle or muscle strain, as well as certain types of headaches and menstrual cramps.

Steroids are also used for inflammation, but in daily clinical practice, NSAIDs are recommended far more routinely for pain than steroids. There are special circumstances in which steroids can also be used for pain, such as when a more pronounced inflammatory process or flare-up is occurring and it is advantageous to get ahead of the inflammatory cascade. NSAIDs typically have fewer side effects than steroids. However, there are cautions about which you should be aware. First, NSAIDs are not completely harmless and are not intended for long-term use. NSAIDs can irritate the stomach and intestinal lining, and chronic use can cause ulcers or perforation—a medical emergency that can be fatal.

Further, while small amounts of aspirin taken on a daily basis are cardioprotective, ibuprofen, naproxen, and certain prescription NSAIDs can increase the risk of heart attack, stroke, and heart failure. Even taking them a few days can increase risk, so it is important to speak with your physician before using them if you have cardiac issues.

One mistake to avoid is determining what amount of over-the-counter NSAIDs is the "prescription dose" and self-prescribing that amount. This is a potentially dangerous practice. The reason the medication is restricted by prescription at higher doses is because people have to be monitored for side effects. They could also unknowingly cause harm from extended use or take too much of the medication.

For instance, 800 mg of ibuprofen is a prescription-strength dose of ibuprofen and is available in a single pill. Knowing that, you might self-prescribe that amount using four 200 mg pills.

However, the surface area of those four pills is actually larger than the surface area of one 800 mg pill, even though their active ingredient content is the same. This means a larger amount of the medication would come in contact with the lining of the stomach or intestines, thus creating a greater chance of stomach irritation, ulceration, or perforation. Available research suggests that roughly 3,200 to 16,500 deaths occur annually from NSAID-related gastrointestinal bleeding.[2] Other statistics reveal that there are 15.3 deaths per 100,000 NSAID users, with up to one-third of those deaths occurring from low-dose aspirin use.[3] Research shows that the number of fatalities from NSAIDs is roughly the same as from opioid medication use. This doesn't undermine the risks involved with opioids, but it does highlight the need for physician oversight and caution even with medication that is generally regarded as benign.

With all of this discussion about side effects and dangerous potential outcomes, you may wonder if we recommend medication at all. Absolutely, we do! However, no medication is completely safe and without risks, so it is important that you understand what constitutes safe use, especially when it comes to OTC medications that aren't prescribed or monitored by a physician.

When acetaminophen and NSAIDs are taken with precautions in mind, they are very effective in not only treating acute pain but also preventing the need for opioid medications, and even preventing the progression to chronic pain. New research has shown that this is especially true when acetaminophen and NSAIDs are used in combination.[4]

One of the ways researchers determine effectiveness in treating pain is by monitoring pain levels after an operation or a procedure and evaluating responses to the pain medication given. What has been found is that the combination of single-dose acetaminophen and single-dose ibuprofen is significantly more effective in reducing postoperative pain compared to single-dose oxycodone, an opioid.[5] This finding translates to everyday pain as well and challenges not only the way we may think of treating acute pain and preventing it from progressing to chronic pain but also the way we may think of treating acute flare-ups in those suffering from chronic pain.

Opioids

As we've discussed, opioids are another class of medications often used to manage pain. Examples of opioid medications include morphine and codeine, among numerous others, but the earliest example is opium, which has been used for thousands of years to treat pain. Opioid medications work primarily by altering the way pain is sensed in the brain but also by altering how the body sends and modulates the pain signal. While opioids can be effective in treating pain, there are inherent risks for addiction and even death. As a result, these medications are available by prescription only and face increasing regulation due to the current opioid epidemic.

Adjuvant Analgesics

Adjuvant analgesics are another group of medications used to treat pain. These are drugs that are usually used to manage conditions other than pain but have been found to work well with certain types of pain too. Some adjuvant analgesics are used to manage neuropathic pain, which is pain caused by altered function, disease, or injury in the nerves, the spinal cord, or the brain. Typically, nerve pain is associated with diabetic neuropathy, nerve compression, shingles, herniated discs, and spinal cord injuries, among other conditions.

The first major group of adjuvant analgesics used in the medical management of neuropathic pain is antidepressant medications. As the name of this class of medications implies, these medications were originally developed to aid in the treatment of depression, but some have been effective in treating certain types of pain, such as neuropathic or nerve pain, various types of headaches, back or pelvic pain, and fibromyalgia. Interestingly, the exact mechanisms of how these medications work are still being researched, but what is known is that they act in the central nervous system, improving depression and reducing pain. Recall that, in the pain pathway, there is an ascending pathway from the body to the spinal cord and the brain and a descending pathway from the brain to the body. It is thought that antidepressants, by increasing norepinephrine and serotonin levels, act on the descending pathway to modulate or reduce pain.

There are three main types of antidepressant medications used for pain. One type, tricyclic medications, has been well researched and is often considered a first-line treatment for nerve pain, including diabetic neuropathy, shingles, peripheral neuropathy, and radiculopathy. The primary example of a tricyclic medication is amitriptyline, but there are several others.

A second type of antidepressant used for pain is serotonin-norepinephrine reuptake inhibitors, or SNRIs. SNRIs are also effective in treating nerve-type pain and have fewer side effects. Two SNRIs, duloxetine and milnacipran, are FDA approved for the treatment of fibromyalgia.

A third type of antidepressant commonly used to manage pain is selective serotonin reuptake inhibitors, or SSRIs. SSRIs don't treat pain per se, but help with functioning and coping. They are especially helpful in improving depression that may be occurring with pain, therefore leading to an increased level of daily functioning and coping.

In general, there are a few important facts to know about antidepressants in regard to the treatment of pain. First, they don't act as quickly as acetaminophen, ibuprofen, or opioids. Rather, these medications take time to reach full effect—sometimes weeks. Also, some antidepressants, especially the tricyclics, have a more pronounced side-effect profile. Thus, they are started at low doses and increased slowly over time in order for doctors to monitor and minimize those effects.

Those taking tricyclics, in particular, need to be closely monitored for drowsiness, disruptive thinking, nausea, weight gain, blurred vision, dry mouth, constipation, difficulty urinating, heart dysrhythmia, and orthostatic hypotension. With SNRIs and SSRIs, side effects occur much less frequently, but a similar list of side effects is monitored that may also include insomnia and increased blood pressure. It is important to note that all antidepressants may increase the risk of suicidal thoughts or actions, so please be sure to speak to your physician or other health-care provider immediately if these occur.

The second major group of adjuvant analgesics is antiepileptic medications. Primary medications include gabapentin and pregabalin. These medications were originally developed to help people who suffer from seizure disorders but were subsequently found to be one of the best options for treating specific types of nerve pain because of their nerve-calming effect. While not FDA approved in this capacity, they also can have an antianxiety effect.

Gabapentin and pregabalin are mostly well tolerated but can cause dizziness, drowsiness, and swelling in the legs and feet. To minimize these side effects, patients generally start with a low dose and slowly increase it. They slowly decrease the dose if discontinuing use.

There are several second- and third-line adjuvant analgesics used for neuropathic pain, including muscle relaxants, baclofen, clonidine, ketamine, and cannabinoids. The potential risks and benefits of using these medications need to be discussed with a physician.

Muscle relaxants are very commonly prescribed to treat musculoskeletal pain and, in particular, low-back pain. However, there is limited and inconsistent research to support their widespread use. A review of available research concluded, "Muscle relaxants have some limited use for acute low-back pain, but the effect is small and the risks of abuse are real. No studies support long term use."[6] The concern is that the occurrence of sedation, drowsiness, dizziness, and other side effects is significant, and the therapeutic benefit may not outweigh these risks. This is especially a consideration if a patient also uses an opioid for the management of pain, as the combined use can cause respiratory suppression that could cause death.

Nonsystemic Approaches

Once again, we are not taking the position that all medications are bad and that you should stop using them. Strategic and thoughtful use of medication can help you have less pain and increase your ability to perform life's daily activities. However, because most analgesics are taken orally, their effects are systemic. In other words, all medications that you take by mouth are absorbed by the gut, go into your bloodstream, and are distributed throughout your entire body. This is one of the primary reasons people may develop the side effects described earlier.

One strategy to optimize the effect of a medication while limiting its systemic side effects is to use it topically over the area of pain instead of taking it by mouth. Some primary examples of this are lidocaine and capsaicin creams or patches, especially when used for neuropathic-type pain. While these have side effects of their own, they are usually prepared so that the analgesic effect is isolated to the area of application as opposed to the entire body.

Lidocaine patches are adhesive patches containing numbing medication that are placed on the site causing pain. The medication is absorbed through the skin and soft tissues to decrease pain. These work well if the stimulus that is causing pain still remains and the pain is not caused by sensitization. Also, the area that is causing pain needs to be superficial enough that the medication can reach the desired target. Painful areas deep inside the body may not respond to a lidocaine patch. This is not a treatment to which you can develop a tolerance, so increasing the dosage strength is not required.[7] Lidocaine patches should not be used by people with severe liver disease or who are taking medication for an arrhythmia. The patches can irritate the skin, so a twelve-hour period of wearing a patch should be followed by twelve hours with it off.

Topical medications are not limited to lidocaine and capsaicin. In fact, there are many other types of patches. Some fairly sophisticated pharmacies can also make many of the NSAIDs and adjuvant analgesics listed above into topical creams. What is nice about these compounds is that you can address multiple sites along the pain pathway with one cream, optimizing local pain control. Again, a key consideration is how deeply the medication can penetrate into the tissues. In other words, these medications need to be able to reach the pain generators within the body. They also need to be absorbed into the skin before clothes can be worn over them.

Noninvasive Modalities

Most interventions for pain, whether medication, manipulation, or an injection, are ultimately about providing neuromodulation, or altering nerve activity to normalize tissue function. This means that to be effective, the treatment must access and normalize as many points along the pain pathway as necessary in order to alter the pain message and minimize the sensation of pain. Noninvasive modalities are an excellent way to alter the pain message and effectively treat pain with fewer side effects.

Cold and heat therapy have long been used for the treatment of pain, though their effectiveness is sometimes overlooked. An advantage is that they are inexpensive and readily available interventions that can work very well for pain. But when and how do you use them? Ice is typically used in the context of acute injuries, when inflammation is the main reason for having pain. But because ice also has a numbing effect that alters the pain message, it can be used for both acute and chronic conditions. There are many differing opinions about when and how often to use ice, but here are a few guidelines. First, it is important to protect your skin, so wrap the ice pack in a thin dish towel or pillowcase. Second, applying ice for fifteen minutes every four hours is an effective dosing strategy to help interrupt the inflammation cycle.

The application of heat is also effective in modulating pain. Heat helps increase blood flow to a painful area and can help soothe and loosen tight muscles, tissues, and joints. In fact, using heat prior to a stretching program can help reduce pain and be an effective strategy to change the strain pattern that is causing chronic pain. However, heat should be avoided in the context of acute injuries. While the increase in blood flow can feel good while the warmth is being applied, it also draws more of the inflammatory cells to the area. So later on, after the heat has been removed, a person can have increased swelling, stiffness, and pain because of the increased inflammation. For this reason, heat is better used for chronic conditions, where inflammation is less of an issue. Again, wrapping the heat source with thin material should protect the skin, and applying heat for fifteen minutes every four hours should be adequate and safe.

Whether using heat or cold treatment, be certain not to use the applications at their extremes or to overdo it. It is normal for the skin to become slightly more pink or flushed with the application of these modalities, but if the tissues become deep red or purple, or if there is increased swelling or blisters, skin damage may have occurred and may need medical attention.

One of the more classic examples of neuromodulation is done through transcutaneous electrical nerve stimulation, or TENS, unit devices. TENS units used to require prescriptions and had to be obtained through pharmacies, physical therapy, or specialty medical supply stores, but they are now FDA approved to be purchased over the counter. There are several different theories about how TENS units work. It is generally accepted that sending electrical nerve stimulation through pads on the skin can alter how the nociceptive message is sent to the spinal cord, thus altering the sensation of pain in the brain.

The stimulation impulses generated by these devices have become quite sophisticated, and animal research studies have shown that TENS can produce opioid peptides that originate internally in the body. As a result, this is a safe way to utilize opioid receptors in the body to reduce pain and increase analgesic effects.[8] TENS units and the theory behind them have led to even more sophisticated devices that can be implanted in the body and apply stimulation directly to the spinal cord. These spinal cord stimulators are discussed in the next section.

Invasive Procedures

For certain types of pain, sometimes medication and noninvasive modalities aren't enough to provide adequate relief. Oftentimes, procedures ranging from soft tissue injections to joint injections to peripheral nerve blocks are indicated. Some types of pain may require even more invasive measures, including epidural injections, plexus and ganglion blocks, spinal cord stimulators, and intrathecal devices.

Soft tissue and joint injections, though considered invasive, are relatively safe and fairly routine when treating common disorders related to musculoskeletal problems or nerve pain, and they often can bring a fair amount of relief and help restore function. One of the main benefits of these injections, if used strategically by a physician, is that they can interrupt or lessen the pain cycle so that structural issues that are contributing to the problem can be more fully addressed.

Soft tissue injections are often used for chronic headaches. Manipulation can then be used to address the structural component causing the headaches. The nerve groups from the upper part of the neck and at the base of the skull sometimes contribute to the generation of certain types of headaches, as these nerves are often compressed by tight muscles. These tight muscles can be considered to be held in relative spasm, and trigger-point injections are injected into key places within the muscles. The injected medication causes the muscles to relax, allowing a physician to then stretch and lengthen the muscles to take pressure off the nerves that are causing the headaches. The use of injections without stretching the muscles is a missed opportunity to make structural changes that may provide pain relief.

Joint injections are a way to control pain when the pain resides in a specific joint. This option is usually for people who suffer from joint arthritis or inflammation. By controlling the amount of inflammation, the symptom of pain is reduced. Typically, the medications that are used are lidocaine, an anesthetic that temporarily blocks the pain message, and a steroid, an anti-inflammatory. Results are variable and can depend on the amount of degeneration within the joint and other contributing factors. The primary risk factors are infection from the procedure, which should be minimized by clean technique, and a short-term increase in blood glucose levels for up to a week. For patients with diabetes, this is an important consideration that must be weighed with a doctor. Generally, a person should not receive more than three steroid injections over the course of a year.

These types of injections can sometimes be very effective in interrupting the pain cycle, but they don't heal the problem. For instance, a knee that has limited joint space or is bone-on-bone will continue to have the same problem. However, injections can allow a person to remain more active and can be used strategically in conjunction with manual treatment or physical therapy to optimize the motion of the joint during a time when the pain is minimized. In some cases, injections can buy a person time to make life changes, such as weight loss, that may improve the function of the joint. In other cases, a joint injection may simply provide some level of comfort until the opportunity for surgery arises.

Nerve blocks are a different type of injection. These are provided more often at the specialty level in medicine, as they are a little less routine and, at times, more invasive. With nerve blocks, a specific nerve has typically been identified, either through physical exam or diagnostic measures, as being the main contributor in the generation of pain. By injecting an anesthetic medication around the nerve, sometimes along with a steroid medication, the pain message is "blocked." Sometimes interrupting that message for an extended period of time can in itself be therapeutic. Other times the block may need to be repeated from time to time as long as it safely provides pain relief for the person. In the headache example mentioned earlier, blocking the nerve that is sending the pain message in addition to injecting and lengthening the muscles that are causing the compression may be helpful.

Facet blocks are another example of nerve blocks. Facets are the joints between individual vertebrae within the spine, and chronic compression of these joints can often lead to chronic pain. Facet blocks can be used, first, to evaluate and confirm if specific joints are the pain generators. If the pain goes away after blocking with a numbing medication, the procedure confirms that site as the one causing pain. The procedure can then be repeated with a slightly different technique called nerve ablation. With nerve ablation, a portion of the nerve sending the pain signal is safely destroyed. This procedure can be used to provide extended relief if it is determined that those specific nerves are sending the pain message from the facet joints.

Epidural injections are often used for a type of pain generated from the neck or back called radicular pain. Radicular pain is pain that radiates from its origin to a distant site. In this case, pain in the arms or legs is caused by the compression of nerve roots coming out of the neck or back. With radicular pain, specific nerve roots coming off the spinal cord are compressed by narrowed vertebral openings, by bulging or herniated discs, or by inflamed surrounding tissue. This type of pain is usually felt as a shooting or traveling pain or numbness in the arms or legs. Sometimes epidural injections can provide relief in these circumstances.

Other times corrective surgery needs to be considered if numbness or radicular pain becomes progressively worse, if the symptoms begin to present with muscle weakness, or if symptoms develop in both limbs. There are some circumstances in which radicular symptoms are considered a surgical emergency. Red-flag symptoms include numbness in the inner thighs and groin area and bowel or bladder function changes, such as a loss of control or an inability to go to the bathroom.

Plexus and ganglion blocks, targeting either nerve network centers or nerve "clusters," are another advanced technique provided by medical specialists. They require a high degree of procedural precision and therefore are considered more invasive. Sympathetic—or fight, flight, or freeze—nerve fibers are targeted in ganglion blocks. These types of blocks are usually considered if abnormal sympathetic messages are contributing to the pain problem, such as with complex regional pain syndrome.

Spinal cord stimulators and intrathecal devices are two more types of invasive interventions. These are considered among the most invasive and specialized pain interventions and are often reserved for painful conditions that have not been responsive to medications and other measures to control pain. Sometimes these are used after surgical procedures have not alleviated pain.

Spinal cord stimulators, as stated previously, use the same type of neuromodulation as TENS units, but the device is placed under the skin; the electrical impulses are applied directly beside the spinal cord. Failed back surgery syndrome, complex regional pain syndrome, radicular pain, and diabetic neuropathy are among the conditions treated with spinal cord stimulators.

The selection criteria for good candidates for spinal cord stimulators are evolving, as research is ongoing. In some cases, a psychiatric evaluation is needed to ensure that a patient will be able to tolerate an implanted device. This is also the case for intrathecal devices.

Intrathecal devices are also implantable devices, but instead of providing spinal cord stimulation, these devices deliver medication, typically an opioid or other highly specialized medication, directly into the space between the spinal cord and the protective sheath that surrounds the spinal cord through a catheter that extends from the device. The use of intrathecal devices is generally reserved for patients with uncontrolled pain conditions, including those who still have pain despite the use of oral opioid pain medications. The goal is to minimize the side effects of oral opioids, such as constipation, sedation, and impaired breathing. By delivering the medication directly near specific areas of the spinal cord, there are fewer systemic effects, and the person has less pain and increased functioning.

This overview of traditional approaches to pain management is not meant to be taken as medical advice. Here are the takeaway points. First, remember that pain medications are used for the purpose of either decreasing the perception of pain in the brain or in the messaging network in the nervous system or blocking the production of specific chemicals that may cause pain within the body. Second, while these approaches often provide some measure of relief, none of them is without its own set of risks or side effects, and so they must be carefully considered and monitored.

Third, pain is individualized and unique. In addition, we have unique body chemistries and structural differences. Therefore, medical treatments also need to be unique and carefully considered. The bottom line is that your treatment plan must be specific for you, your needs, and your situation.

Finally, remember that pain relief is rarely a single-fix solution, a point often missed by both physicians and patients. Sometimes pain is caused by structural problems, not medical ones, and those issues need to be addressed in a structural way. And because pain has mental and emotional components, they have to be considered too. Pain is most effectively treated by accessing as many points as necessary along the pain pathway to make the marginal gains that add up to greater pain relief.

11

Change Your Structure, Change Your Pain

Radical acceptance is to know that painful things are still going to happen, but how we respond makes a difference. We don't have to condone our current reality, but we have to accept it for what it is instead of staying stuck, wishing it were different.

Naomi Judd

In the previous chapter, we discussed the traditional approaches to pain: medical management, noninvasive modalities, and invasive procedures. But as stated before, not every instance of pain has a cause that can be treated with medicine, injection, or surgery. Many times the cause is a musculoskeletal problem that can be addressed only with a structural or functional intervention.

The musculoskeletal system provides the framework in which all other body systems reside and operate. The rib cage houses the heart and lungs, the brain is protected within the head, the spinal cord resides in a canal in the vertebrae, and the gastrointestinal system is suspended within the abdomen. The bones of the skeleton provide anchor and leverage points for the muscles, allowing for movement and locomotion, and in between the muscles are passageways through which blood vessels, nerves, and lymphatic vessels traverse.

In addition, extensive cross-wiring occurs at the spinal-cord level between the musculoskeletal system and the internal body. Therefore, the musculoskeletal system plays a contributing, if not prominent, role in the overall function of the body. If the internal body is not functioning well, this is reflected in the muscles and external body and vice versa. All of these factors affect the body's ability to function normally.

The concept that structure affects function and function affects structure is a key one when it comes to understanding and managing pain. Pain can impact all areas of how we function. It can influence muscle tone and alter the way we move. It can influence breathing and alter heart rate. It can cause the release of stress-response hormones and have a significant impact on how our bodies, organs, and even cells work. Many types of pain are caused by structural changes or functional deficits, affecting life overall. Where we often miss the mark as medical professionals in managing pain is by treating only the symptom of pain without also addressing the underlying structural or functional problems. If those problems are not properly addressed, the symptom of pain will likely not improve.

Margaret's Story

To better understand how problems in the musculoskeletal system can affect pain and overall health, consider Margaret.[1] Margaret, a thirty-eight-year-old high school business and economics teacher, had a minor car accident in which she was rear-ended by another driver. Margaret had forcefully slammed on her brakes to avoid the car in front of her, but the driver behind her noticed too late that traffic was coming to an abrupt stop. Upon impact, she sustained a mild whiplash-type injury to her neck, and her rib cage was compressed by the seat belt. Though the accident wasn't severe enough to deploy her airbags, the next day she had mild pain in her neck, shoulders, and low back.

In the weeks that followed, Margaret developed headaches and nausea and wasn't able to generate much of an appetite. She dropped her exercise routine because she felt restricted in her breathing, like she couldn't get a full breath. Her symptoms began to affect her sleep, and her concentration during the day began to suffer. Lesson plans and classroom teaching became more of a chore, and she was more irritable with her husband and ten-year-old daughter. She felt all "torqued up." It seemed as if her minor accident was beginning to affect everything in her life.

Several factors contributed to the domino effect of pain and dysfunction in her life. At the heart of it was the impact itself. During the accident, Margaret was in a seated position with her right leg fully extended, pressing fully against the brake pedal, and her arms braced against the steering wheel. With the heavy braking, her seat belt locked against her waist and rib cage to hold her in place. And then there was the impact. All the kinetic energy of the vehicle behind her was transferred through her body in the strained position she was seated in, and the normal postural and gravitational strain patterns in her muscles and fascia were immediately changed. This impact changed the tension length of her muscles and fascia; it changed the orientation of the joints in her pelvis, back, and neck; and her rib cage was now restricted. The nerves at the base of her skull were compressed, leading to nausea and headaches. It is no wonder she felt "torqued up."

Structural, Not Medical

The types of problems Margaret experienced won't go away with ibuprofen, though it can help with inflammation that might occur.

They won't go away with muscle relaxants, though they might help in the short term with any associated muscle spasm. And opioids will do little to address the underlying issues and will open the risk for addiction. Simply stated, Margaret had a structural problem, not primarily a medical one.

Addressing pain from a structural standpoint is vital. To understand this, let's consider Margaret's issues one by one. Her initial neck pain is perhaps the most direct piece to understand. During the impact from behind, Margaret's neck likely extended back toward her headrest and then flexed forward toward her chest. This action may have stretched the ligaments and tissues in the front and back of her neck. If she was looking in the mirror slightly to the right to see if a car was heading toward her, the impact occurred in an asymmetrical way. This created dysfunction in the movement and orientation of her neck, which can cause pain. Further, with even a mild strain, there can be an inflammatory response, and the muscles of the neck might go into spasm reflexively to stabilize or "splint" the neck to prevent further injury. This persistent muscle spasm creates a buildup of lactic acid in the muscles, which irritates nerves, and with decreased blood flow through the spasming muscles, there is a relative lack of oxygen in these tissues. These factors can contribute to pain as well.

Margaret's headaches were likely caused by two separate factors. The more obvious contributor may be the spasm in the neck muscles that compresses nerves at the base of the skull and near attachments at the bony prominences behind the ears, causing pain that can radiate over the top of and around the head. However, some of her headaches could also be due to dysfunction of her neck vertebrae, as some headache pain follows very specific referral patterns based on where nerves originate at different levels within the neck. The nausea likely had similar causes. One of the main nerves that controls the autonomic activity of the stomach, the vagus nerve, exits from the base of the skull. Compression of that nerve from muscle spasm or tissue congestion from inflammation can disrupt the normal functional activity of the stomach, causing nausea.

Margaret's back pain was likely caused by the position of her body during the accident. She was seated and therefore in a flexed position, and she was pressing hard on the brake pedal. This created asymmetry in her back, pelvis, and sacroiliac joints. And then the impact occurred. This immediately created a new, abnormal strain pattern within these structures. Asymmetry can lead to compressive forces within any of these joints and lead to pain and discomfort.

The difficulty Margaret developed with breathing and getting a full breath likely had two causes. The most obvious cause was the compression of the rib cage from the seat belt, which limited the movement of the rib cage. The second cause was related to the diaphragm, which drives breathing and is anchored at the bottom of the rib cage. Likely, the impact of the accident affected the movement of this muscle, and if it became tight and restricted, as any muscle can, it restricted her breathing.

Margaret's story demonstrates several points. First, it demonstrates how structural factors contribute to overall discomfort and pain levels. Second, it shows that while a short course of anti-inflammatory medications and muscle relaxants would certainly help alleviate inflammation and muscle spasm, they would do little to address the abnormal strain patterns in the body that contribute to ongoing problems. These are structural problems that require structural solutions.

The Relationship between Structure and Function

Now let's look at how abnormal relationships between structure and function can create problems in the *absence* of injury, as was the case for Anna.[2] Anna was fourteen years old and suffered from headaches, discomfort between her shoulders, and low-back pain. She had a slumped posture, carrying her head a fair amount ahead of her shoulders, and her pelvis tucked underneath her body. Her siblings would tease that she had no bottom, and her parents often reminded her to stand up straight. Her parents assumed, correctly, that poor posture contributed to her headaches and low-back pain. However, no measure of gentle chiding or genuine effort on Anna's part seemed to correct the problem.

Further questioning revealed that she always woke up fatigued and her headaches were worse in the morning. In addition to the abnormalities noted in her posture, other abnormalities were found in her physical exam, specifically the ear, nose, and throat exam. There was a deviated septum in her nose, a thickening of the mucosa in the inside of her cheeks, and gapping of her front teeth even when her jaw was closed. Her tongue was also coated with a white film. These were all signs that Anna was having difficulty breathing through her nose at night.

In fact, Anna had difficulty breathing through her nose at all, but at night it was nearly impossible. Sheepishly, Anna confessed that she'd been told she had a bit of a snoring problem. Her postural changes were largely compensatory efforts to open her oral and nasal passageways at night. Snoring occurs when the air passageways are narrowed or congested, and a person has to breathe through the mouth to overcome the deficit in air movement.

In addition, Anna probably needed to flex her head forward to draw the tongue, which should rest at the top of the palate, away from the posterior portion of the throat, where it was narrowing the air passage. If the tongue isn't resting against the top of the palate, it has to go somewhere. To pull the tongue away from the back of the throat, a person unconsciously presses it forward into the teeth. Over time, this pushes the teeth forward and the person develops a need for braces. Or the person bites the inside of their cheeks to make space between their upper and lower teeth for their tongue. All of this occurs to keep the air passageways open.

So what does this have to do with pain? The forward flexion of the head, which occurs nightly for six to eight hours, can create a slumped posture in the neck and upper back. Because this is a less efficient posture, pain can develop in the neck, back, and low back. In addition, it can cause headaches because of the postural strain on the nerves that provide sensation to the head and scalp. Furthermore, because people with sleep-disturbed breathing are not getting enough oxygen at night, they wake up with headaches, not feeling refreshed in the morning because their sleep wasn't restorative—they are working all night to breathe! This exacerbates any latent postural problem and lowers the threshold for pain to occur.

So the back pain, neck pain, and headaches were the result of the functional problem of sleep-disturbed breathing. A person cannot treat symptoms of a functional problem simply by trying to stand up straighter or by taking ibuprofen. A functional problem requires a functional solution, and the pain will improve as a consequence of improved function just the same way it began as a result of compromised function.

Addressing the Source beyond the Symptoms

With both Margaret and Anna, the areas in pain were not the root problem. And while medication may have perhaps helped reduce some of the symptoms, it would not effectively address the underlying problems. They required something different.

Margaret was referred to an osteopathic physician to be evaluated for structural dysfunction. Osteopathic physicans are fully licensed doctors that can provide manual treatment in addition to medical management and surgery. The doctor provided a full orthopedic and neurologic exam and obtained X-rays to ensure there were no spinal injuries. She provided osteopathic manipulative treatment (OMT), using a series of gentle manipulative techniques to remove compressive forces and restore normal movement in the joints and to reduce muscle spasm in the neck, upper shoulder, and back regions. Restoring motion in the neck vertebrae and decreasing the muscular tension at the base of the skull alleviated the referred headaches and nausea after only a couple of treatments. Care was also taken to remove the restriction at the thoracolumbar portion of her back, where both the hip flexors and abdominal diaphragm are anchored. This not only allowed her to get a deeper breath but also allowed her to feel like she could exercise again. After five treatments with OMT, most of her symptoms had resolved.

Anna also sought care from an osteopathic physician, but here the focus was optimizing her breathing function and correcting her structural issues with OMT. The doctor first addressed how Anna slept at night and took steps to minimize her snoring. A non-habit-forming nasal spray containing xylitol and saline was suggested. This helped decongest the nasal tissues at night and increase airflow. Anna was also instructed to wear external nasal strips or internal nasal dilators to increase the size of the air passageways at night.

Anna was also referred to a dentist and a physical therapist who specialized in myofunctional retraining to address the misalignment of her teeth and to provide exercises that created awareness of the facial muscles and the muscles of the mouth. The goal was to correct the factors that caused sleep-disordered breathing and to retrain the muscles of the tongue, mouth, and throat to reduce obstruction of the airway. Six months later, after compliance with all aspects of her care, things gradually began to change for Anna. She was more upright, her posture had improved dramatically, and many of her oral symptoms had gone away. She was not oxygen deprived at night, so she woke up refreshed and without headaches. While she had been a good student before treatment, she was able to have more stamina and focus at school.

We could offer numerous examples to show how a functional deficit creates the symptom of pain. The point is that when pain is the result of functional deficit, the restoration of normal function is often the best option to reduce pain. Pills do not restore function, and if they are the only method used for treatment, there is less chance for resolution of pain because the root cause is not being addressed. With pain, just as with any problem in life, one has to recognize the underlying issues in order to rectify it. If the underlying issues are not addressed, symptoms may be partially alleviated, but the problem will not go away.

The Benefits of Manipulation as Treatment

Manipulation can provide many physiologic benefits that can be helpful in treating pain. We discussed earlier that manipulation can help with nociceptive, mechanical pain in which compressive forces affect joints. Joints that are compressed are likely to develop osteoarthritic changes over time because of altered blood flow, decreased oxygen and nutrition to the joint, and impaired cellular function. Restoring normal joint mechanics can help keep joints mobile and healthy. Even joints that do have arthritic changes can benefit from better mobility.

Furthermore, manipulation affects the nerve-messaging signals from the body to the spinal cord. In other words, it can interrupt and change the pain messaging sent to the brain. This can be accomplished by decreasing tissue swelling, muscle restriction, and nerve compression. It can also improve blood supply and venous and lymphatic drainage from an area, thereby improving cellular nutrition and metabolism of the structures involved.

Manipulation can restore normal muscle length in dysfunctional strain patterns, altering local sensitization and decreasing tender points within fascia and muscles. All of this helps reduce chronic pain. Remember, if chronic pain develops because of neuroplasticity in one direction, every effort should be made to use the power of neuroplasticity in the other direction to restore normal function.

But why has it taken so long for structural approaches to receive acceptance in the medical community, while patients have been seeing those who provide manipulation in droves for decades? Some of the difficulty lies in the challenges of putting manipulative approaches through research the same way one would when evaluating the efficacy of a new medication. First, the best of these types of studies are double-blind studies, meaning that neither the physician nor the patient knows if the patient is receiving the actual medication or a placebo. This is difficult to accomplish with manipulation because the physician who provides the manipulation or the manipulation placebo cannot be blind to it. Second, the application of manipulation, whether from an MD, a DO, a chiropractor, or a physical therapist, can be vastly different and, moreover, highly operator-dependent. In other words, just as with surgeons, there can be a vastly different skill set from one person who provides manipulation compared to the next, even when performing the same or similar techniques.

Still, there is some very good research providing support for manipulative care. Outcome studies, as opposed to randomized, double-blind clinical trials, are often used to study the benefits of manipulation and to evaluate clinical and cost-effectiveness analysis. These studies can help provide an understanding of the successful, replicable interventions. In the case of spinal manipulation, outcome studies prove to be highly favorable. Outcomes from random controlled trials[3] provide "grade A" evidence that spinal manipulation achieves pain reduction, earlier return to work, shortened disability and impairment, less medication use, fewer physical therapy visits, and increased patient satisfaction.[4]

As more physicians and practitioners seek out this training, and as additional studies demonstrate cost-effective benefit for people who suffer from chronic pain, manipulation will be well positioned to provide a safe option in addition to traditional medical treatment for pain. But how do you know what type of manipulation is best for you, and whose care should you seek? Referral from a primary care physician is often a good place to start. Your physician will most likely know which colleagues provide effective manipulation in the community or can ask other physicians and patients. Online reviews can be helpful, especially if there are enough reviews to provide a clear picture of overall patient satisfaction. You also might be able to get an idea of techniques used, whether the techniques are gentle, and if patients had good success. If you decide on a provider, you should call the office to ask about credentials. When calling physicians' offices, ask if they are residency trained or board certified in the services they offer. For chiropractors or physical therapists, ask for the name of the college where they received their training and what additional credentials they have attained. Finally, word of mouth is a great way to find someone with the skill set you need. If people are getting results, or if they aren't, they will share it.

🌰

It is important to remember that pain often has a structural component as a contributing root for its cause. If the major underlying problem is structural, this will not be corrected with medication alone. Addressing structural restrictions or dysfunction in the hands of a skilled physician, chiropractor, or manual practitioner can provide an important marginal gain in the process of reducing pain, often with few, if any, side effects. Make certain you look into changing your structure to change your pain.

12

Change Your Beliefs, Change Your Pain

People who pray for courage, for strength to bear the unbearable, for the grace to remember what they have left instead of what they have lost, very often find their prayer answered.

Harold S. Kushner

I (Linda) am a member of a Presbyterian church. Every Sunday we recite a creed that states what we believe. Some people find this exercise rote and boring. To me, it is meaningful, as it continues to reinforce the tenets of my faith. It causes me to pause and think, *What do I believe, and do I really believe what I am saying? Are these core beliefs, beliefs I can stand behind? Do I guide my life by these principles? Do my life experiences support these beliefs?*

This type of self-reflection on what we believe is important because our thoughts, feelings, and behaviors are generated from our beliefs. Our beliefs have everything to do with how we see the world and how we interpret things. For example, if you believe people can't be trusted, you will have negative thoughts, emotions, and behaviors based on that belief. If you believe people can be trusted, you will have positive thoughts, emotions, and behaviors based on that belief. We all hold beliefs about the world, our lives, and even pain.

Our beliefs are often formed in childhood through interactions with our original families and others. They can also be formed by traumatic events, injuries, or the presence of chronic pain. Basically, our life experiences, accompanied by the voices of those around us and our own interpretation of events, form our beliefs. But we are not victims of our experiences. We can change the way we interpret them.

Throughout our lives, we are constantly evaluating situations either to reinforce our current beliefs or to change them. Most of the time, we are unwilling to give up our beliefs unless we have a great deal of evidence to the contrary. Beliefs, as compared to thoughts, are more resistant to change. The more history we have with a belief, the more we hang on to it. Still, we can change our beliefs.

While our beliefs might not be written down on a piece of paper, they are a script running in our heads, playing out the movie of our lives. Whether conscious or unconscious, our beliefs impact our reactions to pain. They can prompt our behaviors, contribute to our distress and decreased activity, and lead to feeling helpless. Or they can spur us on, help us find meaning in our pain, and turn down the volume on pain.

Thoughts that come into our heads cannot be separated from our beliefs. The two are entwined. The way we think has a direct and an indirect effect on physical and psychological factors associated with pain. Behind our thoughts are our beliefs. Thus, it is helpful to look at our beliefs concerning pain. Some of those beliefs will help us feel better; others will weigh us down.

Two Mind-Sets

Psychologist Carol Dweck says that there are two types of mind-sets: growth and fixed. Mind-sets are beliefs and attitudes. In her book *Mindset*,[1] she discusses how every aspect of our lives is influenced by how we think. People with a fixed mind-set focus only on success and blame others when they don't reach their goals. They ruminate over their problems, and when they have a setback, they become depressed and tell themselves they are unworthy. They measure themselves by failure.

People with a growth mind-set thrive on challenges and stretch themselves beyond the possible. When they have a setback, they cope by being more determined. They develop a mental toughness. Setbacks are a wake-up call to keep going. They want to improve and grow, not just win.

Living beyond pain is certainly a challenge and requires mental toughness. The view you adopt for yourself with regard to pain will powerfully affect the way you live your life. A fixed mind-set says pain will lead to disability. A growth mind-set says pain might slow you down, but you can adjust, learn new ways to approach pain, and continue to grow as a person. Believing that you can grow and change despite pain will push you forward in life. Beliefs—and other cognitive interpretations that you make about pain—impact everything you think, feel, do, and try to do.

Your communication about your pain with significant others, physicians, coworkers, health-care providers, and others is born out of your beliefs about your pain. When you communicate, you emphasize certain aspects of your pain based on your interpretation. Your perspective rules the day and forms an appraisal. And when that appraisal is negative, it leads to negative thoughts that make pain worse.

Reframing Beliefs toward a Growth Mind-Set

Because beliefs are behind your thoughts, emotions, and behaviors associated with pain, it is helpful to identify them, understand them, and determine if an alternate view regarding pain could move you forward. Do you need to reframe your pain by moving from a fixed to a growth mind-set? Could you see pain as a gift or a symptom that causes you to grow?

We hope your answer is yes, but you may not be convinced that this is possible yet. Right now you may just want the pain to stop and have little interest in finding the good in pain. But what you currently believe about pain is influencing your recovery. So why not spend a little time reflecting on the beliefs that drive you to struggle, survive, or thrive? If you are going to rebuild your life, taking inventory of your pain beliefs can be a helpful exercise.

Here are ten common negative beliefs about pain that can lead to negative thoughts, feelings, and behaviors. The left side of the column represents a fixed mind-set. But notice how it is possible to reframe those beliefs to help you manage pain in a positive way. The right column reflects a growth mind-set. Negative beliefs will keep you stuck. Believing differently will move you forward.

NEGATIVE BELIEF	REFRAMED BELIEF
Nothing can be done to make me better.	If I apply the concept of marginal gains, there are a number of things that can be done to make me better. Just like the British Tour de France team, I can identify the 1 percent change I can make here and there that will add up to not only winning the pain challenge but also growing through it.
I cannot cope with my pain.	I can cope with difficult things. It won't be easy and will probably be a struggle, but I can do it if I put my mind to it. If I have faith, anything is possible.
I have no control.	I have control over my responses to pain. I have control over how I think about pain and will take control where and when I can.
I am not going to make it.	It might be a long and difficult path, but I can make it and will hang on to hope.
Life isn't fair.	Bad things do happen to good people. Life isn't fair, but difficulty challenges me to be a better person.

NEGATIVE BELIEF	REFRAMED BELIEF
My body is defective; it betrays me.	Imperfection is part of being human. It is unrealistic to think my body will never fail in any way. To be human is to be imperfect.
I am not functioning and can't do anything.	Functioning may be compromised for a time, but I can work to a new normal.
I am a burden.	I need extra help right now, but I am working toward more independence.
I am weak.	When I am weak, others, including God, show me their strength, and I can lean on them until I am stronger. With effort, I can get stronger.
I am useless and will be rejected.	While I breathe and live, I have purpose. I am valued and unconditionally loved.

Let's expand on each of these beliefs.

Nothing Can Be Done to Make Me Better

When you are at a point of frustration with chronic pain, it is easy to start believing that all the efforts to feel better seem futile. Opioid medications can numb the pain, but they don't make chronic pain better. As you begin to better understand how chronic pain behaves, you can learn that there is actually quite a bit that can be done to make you feel better. Strategic small changes can add up to a win for living beyond pain.

Joe was completely disabled, gained eighty pounds, developed type 2 diabetes, and could hardly walk. He received disability and was at home watching his life waste away until someone he knew began to believe in him. Joe had been a firefighter prior to his injury, and his friend remembered that man.

With his friend's encouragement, Joe began a very basic Pilates exercise program. At first, he could hardly balance. He fell down constantly and struggled. But his friend refused to give up on Joe because he understood the concept of marginal gains and the growth mind-set. He pushed Joe to do one thing every day in that exercise program. He would not allow Joe to believe that nothing could be done. As Joe slowly and steadily began to move and balance his body, he grew stronger. Joe lost weight and controlled his diabetes through diet. By the end of nine months, Joe was walking and capable of getting a new job. Believing that something could be done helped change his life.

I Cannot Cope with My Pain

When Mary started therapy, she was convinced that she couldn't cope with her pain. "I don't even understand my pain. How do I cope with something I don't even understand? The pain moves to different parts of my body. No one can explain it to me. Some days I feel like I am losing my mind. I am on lots of pills. I need answers because I am this close to giving up."

Mary's pain was real, intense, and causing her to suffer. But the belief that she couldn't cope with it was making it worse. In fact, there were several lifestyle changes Mary could make immediately that would help her cope with her pain. I (Linda) asked Mary to tell me about a difficult challenge in her life that she had overcome. Mary had been through a lot as a child and had overcome tremendous odds to become a successful business owner and mother to three children.

Recalling several stories of her resilience as a child helped her realize that she could cope with difficult things. Pain was now her difficult thing. She had to believe it was the next challenge to overcome. As she began to apply the strategies and changes discussed in this book, Mary soon realized that she could cope with her pain without narcotics and see improvement.

I Have No Control

We have already mentioned that a core struggle with pain is the feeling of being out of control in so many areas of your life. Besides all the health struggles, there are things like social events that create uncertainty because your body may not cooperate and daily tasks that don't get done because they feel overwhelming. Research tells us that our ability to control pain is a significant predictor of health outcomes and improved function.[2] If you believe you have control over your pain, you will do better. As you will learn in a later chapter, the opposite of believing you have control is catastrophic thinking. This type of thinking leads to more pain and feelings of helplessness.

The truth is none of us has control over many things that happen to us in our lives. That said, there are things we can do to take back control in some areas. Feelings of control are enhanced by the belief that we have purpose in life and everything can be used for good in some way. The question is not whether you can cope with out-of-control feelings but whether you can work through them. You need to control the parts of the pain that you can and surrender the rest. For example, say to yourself, "I can't control the suffering I feel sometimes, but I can control how I respond to that suffering. When I control my response, I can impact my suffering in a good way. That is one part of pain I can control." In other words, keep moving forward while accepting the things you can't control.

I Am Not Going to Make It

This belief is a good example of being deceived into thinking life is hopeless. When we give in to hopelessness, we stop believing that we can continue to impact the future by our actions today. We also think that no one understands or will support us. Nothing could be further from the truth. We hope to convey in this book that we, and many others, understand the difficulty of living with chronic pain. Again, with a growth mind-set, chronic pain can be seen as something that can bring self-examination and growth. You are alive and making it, maybe not the way you would like, but that can be addressed. As long as you breathe, you have purpose and value.

Find people who will encourage you through this journey. Those people exist and will support and encourage you if you make efforts to find them. But you have to fight the hopeless thoughts with the truth that nothing is ever hopeless. There is always a glimmer of light, even if it is just a glimmer.

Life Isn't Fair

If you believe life isn't fair because of your pain, that belief will bring anxiety and even anger. You will have no peace focusing on the injustice of experiencing pain. In fact, focusing on pain as an unfair experience usually ends in bitterness.

We don't live in an ideal world free from pain and suffering. The creation story reminds us that God created a perfect world that became imperfect due to humanity's sin. Because of that sin, we suffer on this side of heaven. The biblical account of Job is a prime example. The book begins with a statement that Job was a righteous man. It quickly unfolds into a story that seems quite unfair. Job endured tremendous hardship and never knew why he was suffering such pain and loss. Through his pain and hardship, which seemingly came for no reason, Job chose to trust God. Job had a core belief that God was good all the time. His circumstances brought this belief into question. He could have thought, *God has let me down. I don't deserve this.* Instead, he moved through his pain, choosing to trust what didn't make sense because he fundamentally believed in the goodness of God.

I (Linda) have always had an issue with fairness. As the youngest of three, I watched how my brothers were treated whenever they pushed the limits or decided to challenge my dad on a rule. My dad was big on fairness, and being the only girl did not garner me special treatment. Dad gave us whatever we deserved based on our behavior. When we acted out, there was a consequence to pay.

Fairness was such an issue for me that when I became college age, I applied to the University of Michigan with the intent to eventually go to law school. I wanted to be a part of those who championed fairness. But when my oldest brother was blown up on an airplane by a terrorist bomb, life did not seem fair. I lost interest in the law, feeling that nothing could be done to right what I perceived to be a tremendous wrong.

For people in pain, it is common to say or think, "Life isn't fair." Your life feels as if it has blown up. "Why do I have this pain that won't go away?" Like Job, we aren't always privy to definitive answers. When we don't know why, do we allow bitterness to drive our lives? Or do we accept the pain of this world and do our best to reduce or stop it? Do we hang on to our beliefs? Do we maintain a positive mind-set and, like Job, learn through the pain?

My Body Is Defective; It Betrays Me

One of my (Linda's) best friends, Steve, recently received bad news regarding a health diagnosis. He told me, "Pain is a reminder that something is physically wrong with me. And living with that means I have to intentionally fight fear."

Steve's dad died at the age of thirty-nine from arteriosclerosis. This heart disease narrows the arteries due to thickening of the arterial wall. Basically, the normally flexible walls in the arteries harden, restricting blood flow to the organs and tissue. With no knowledge of having heart disease, Steve's dad had a heart attack and died one year later. So when Steve, who is now in his fifties, began having symptoms, he went to his doctor. The diagnosis was the same as his dad's. The pain he was having now had a name. He was told that his pain could be managed, but the disease was not reversible.

When I heard the news, my first thought was, *He didn't choose his heredity!* He has worked hard to live a healthy lifestyle, yet this disease has been silently progressing in his body. His recent pain was like a notification on social media. It brought attention to a problem of which he was unaware. Once he explored the pain, the reality of his disease was made known.

When I asked Steve how he is living with the pain, he told me that the pain has given him a heightened awareness of his body and changes. He is much more aware of his surroundings and how he is living his life. He wanted me to know that when you live with a chronic condition and pain, you have a choice. You can become a victim, feeling as though your body has betrayed you and focusing on its defects, or you can use your values to refuse victim status. Steve has a growth mind-set.

Steve made a choice to be intentional about his life. When fear creeps into his mind, he chooses to move in his faith and trust God for every day, not giving in to the fear. Fear, he reminded me, can be devastating and take you to a place of anxiety and depression. It can lead to avoidance. He doesn't want to go there and will fight to stay positive and intentional. Fear would waste away his happy moments. He has decided not to let his heart be troubled and not to be afraid. He can't change much about his heart health at this point, but he can stand against fear and move away from the belief that he is a victim.

I Am Not Functioning and Can't Do Anything

When chronic pain takes hold, functioning often changes. You have to get used to a new normal, but it is not true that you can't do anything. You may have to do things differently. You may have to slow down or take extra time to readjust. However, you can do things, maybe just not in the way you did before. Avoid thinking in all-or-nothing terms. Saying you can't do anything is based on all-or-nothing thinking.

Life is not lived in black and white. If you don't adjust your expectations and start working on better functioning, resentment will set in. So commit to the concept of marginal gains and persevere to improve your functioning as much as possible. Remember the British team and how every small change made a big difference. Small steps are steps to victory.

I Am a Burden

When someone is disabled by chronic pain, they often worry that they are burdening others around them. Being a burden means you are being carried by others. When you are sick or dealing with pain, others do have to step in and help carry you. But if you consider the big picture, you realize that over time you will begin to take back as much independence as possible.

Problems develop when you don't try to do more for yourself and remain satisfied with a growing dependence on others due to chronic pain. You do burden others if you become emotionally difficult and create stress and worry for them. However, you have the power not to let this happen even if you are in pain.

Most of us are better at taking care of others than allowing others to take care of us. And the reality of our dependence in some areas can be felt when someone makes an insensitive comment. All it might take is a social media post to bring up feelings of inadequacy. When this type of thinking takes hold, you have to fight back with truth. Your life has changed in certain ways, but you are functional and can contribute. You exist. You are valuable. You are here for a reason, and there are things for you to do.

Those momentary feelings of being a burden may come, but they also go. Don't dwell on them. Change your thoughts. You didn't choose to have pain, and you are working hard to get back in the game of life. Your life may look different from before, but you will adjust if you put your mind to it. Saying "Today is not a great day" is how you feel today. Tomorrow can be better.

Sometimes in their zeal to help, family members do too much and reinforce the idea that you are a burden. You may have to tell them to back off now and then. If so, do it with love, knowing their intentions are probably good. Let them know that you need time to adjust and may need to be pushed to try things on your own (within reason, of course). Be sensitive to their time and their care for you; ask if they need a break. Let them know that your desire is to work toward more independence.

I Am Weak

We all have times in our lives when we feel weak due to life circumstances or the buildup of stress. During those times, we are reminded that when we are weak, faith can be a source of strength. In the Bible, the apostle Paul felt weak about something, possibly a physical affliction, that he desperately wanted removed from his life. When the thing was not removed, he concluded that God's grace was sufficient and that God's power was made perfect in his weakness. Instead of becoming bitter, he allowed God to shine through his weakness. This doesn't mean he never struggled with it or that his preference wasn't healing.

In today's culture, weakness is seen as a liability and something that diminishes our value in the eyes of others. However, weakness can become a reminder of the fragility of life and refocus our priorities. We can find strength in weakness. This is how we grow. Physical weakness often reveals a heart of self-reliance and a desire to do things in our own strength. Contentment is found when we realize our weaknesses can be used to renew our inner lives and spirits. We also learn the importance of community in times of trouble and weakness. When we surround ourselves with encouraging people, they can lift us up.

When you feel weak, meditate, pray, and find a friend who can encourage you. Weakness can bring out strength.

I Am Useless and Will Be Rejected

Rebecca suffered for years from low-back pain related to an injury. She was unable to keep up with her daily activities and was fearful that anything she did would result in more pain. Her chronic pain was severe. As a result, she felt useless and worried that people would reject her based on her inability to do very much. Nothing she tried with numerous doctors seemed to work. Clearly, Rebecca's pain had dampened her quality of life. She felt useless most of the time.

The belief of being useless is based on the idea that performance determines worth, a characteristic of a fixed mind-set. If you can no longer do what you used to do because of pain, this does not render you useless. This is all-or-nothing thinking because it doesn't consider new possibilities. Maybe you can't be used in the same ways you were before, but you can do some things. As you accept the limitations that you face, you can also continue to gently push yourself to make marginal gains. Embrace a good day when you can accomplish a few things. Look forward to having those days again. Don't isolate from those who love you. Instead, join in when you are able. Most of all, don't give up hope or define your worth in terms of what you can do.

As we conclude this section, we hope you see that identifying your beliefs regarding pain is important. If those beliefs are negative or extreme (all or nothing), they will lead to negative thoughts, feelings, and behaviors. So begin to challenge those beliefs. Write them down. Ask yourself how strongly you believe them. Then look for evidence to help you reject them. What are better ways to think about your life story? Do you want pain to be in control of your destiny? If not, generate alternative beliefs and chip away at those that support a negative view of life. Begin to develop a growth mind-set.

We challenge you to act to counter a negative belief and see what happens. For example, act as if you are useful. Then notice the difference in how you think and feel. Stop giving negative beliefs so much airtime in your mind. It's time for a more positive approach because the power of the mind can moderate pain. Are you ready to create a more positive mind-set?

13

Change Your Thoughts, Change Your Pain

It's not the situation that's causing your stress, it's your thoughts, and you can change that right here and now. You can choose to be peaceful right here and now. Peace is a choice, and it has nothing to do with what other people do or think.

Gerald G. Jampolsky

When I was in my late forties, I (Linda) took my kids to my hometown ice-skating rink during a Thanksgiving visit to my family in Michigan. Growing up, I was on double-runner skates at the age of four and ice-skated throughout my childhood. We had an outdoor ice-skating rink with a warming house in my neighborhood. Every day after school, I'd walk home, take my skates to the rink, and skate until it was dark or time for dinner. I loved to float on the ice. It was freeing, relaxing, and a way to spend time with friends. Ice-skating is a part of life in the north. It's just something you do!

So when I had a chance to introduce my Virginia-born children to the rink, I was excited. They would experience the joy of ice-skating and see a special part of my childhood. As my young children cautiously made their way on the ice, I skated around them and decided to try a few moves from my childhood, like a flying camel. I flew into the air feeling sixteen years old again but did not make the landing. Instead, I found my fortysomething body flat on the ice and in so much pain that I was scared. I didn't want to frighten my children, so I pretended to be okay, but inside I knew something was seriously wrong. Should I calmly ask my children to find an adult who could call 911? I couldn't move, but I was determined not to traumatize my kids on the ice. Eventually, I was able to get up and walk back to the warming house, but the pain was unbearable.

A few months went by, and the pain worsened to the point that I could not sit or sleep. I could not find a comfortable position and had a few moments of relief only when standing. I tried one opioid pill, but I couldn't tolerate it. It made my head spin and made me dizzy and nauseous—this was worse than the pain. I have a history of being very sensitive to any medication and used to joke with my parents that I would never become an addict because most substances make me feel ill. Opioids were not the answer for me, but if I could have tolerated them, I would have taken them. I remember thinking, *I will do anything to make this pain stop.* And in those days, we were told that opioids were safe to take for chronic pain.

As I searched for ways to relieve the pain, I tried chiropractic care, exercise, stretching, anti-inflammatory pills, and many medical doctors. Nothing brought relief. No one had answers for me. Finally, I found an acupuncture-trained physician who provided me hours of relief at a time. But he noticed how quickly the pain returned and sent me for an MRI, convinced I had a structural problem that could not be fixed with acupuncture. By this time, my pain had been with me for months and was causing me problems even when working in my home office. I began to panic over the unremitting pain I had with no diagnosis.

Had I known what I know now, I would have realized that my thinking process was amplifying my pain. I was completely focused on how much I hurt and how much the pain was impairing me. The pain seemed to grow daily, and my thoughts became more anxious and panic laden. I would think, *I have kids, a husband, a job. I can't go on like this.*

I had a pain story that needed a rewrite. Being at the mercy of my pain had placed me in a victim position, and pain was in control. When I thought about the future, I saw terrible outcomes. In my head, my thoughts were looping like a never-ending cycle of negativity. I saw problems and no solutions.

My negative thinking was making my pain worse. In fact, the more I catastrophized my pain, the more intense it became and the more tired I felt. Catastrophic thoughts are one of the amplifiers of pain. They are like gasoline on a fire. They trip the pain alarm. They lead to feeling helpless.

Fortunately, the acupuncture physician made the right call. The MRI showed the problem—a bulging disc on L5 causing pain to my sciatic nerve. Several doctors recommended a surgical solution, a microdiscectomy. For me, the surgery was a success. (I will come back to this story later regarding the lack of postoperative help.) But my thoughts of doom and gloom had amplified my pain. I had obsessed about my pain and had turned it into something greater than it needed to be. Yes, I hurt terribly, but my catastrophic thinking had made my pain worse.

Because the brain processes both emotional and physical pain, attending to both the physical and the psychological issues involved in pain is necessary. Attending to thoughts of a catastrophic nature is an area to target for change. The less you use this type of thinking, the less suffering you will have. Change your thoughts, change your pain. This is a low-risk, high-benefit way to improve your pain.

Catastrophic Thinking: An Amplifier of Pain

Catastrophic thinking is a strong predictor of pain intensity.[1] It is a way of thinking that is considered a cognitive distortion. It involves seeing an unfavorable outcome, deciding if that outcome will happen, and then deciding that if it does, the results will be a disaster. Basically, it is a negative forecast of future events. When we think negatively about our pain, expect the worst, and magnify our problems, we turn up the volume on pain.

Catastrophic thinking involves ruminating on thoughts such as the following: *This is terrible. The pain will never go away. I can't cope. I can't take it anymore. All I can think about is how much it hurts. Something terrible must be the cause.* Notice the negative predictions about future outcomes that are most likely not realistic. Having this type of mind-set is a predictor of pain intensity, the need for opioid medications, the length of hospital stay after surgery, how well treatments will work, and if someone will become disabled from their pain.[2] That is how powerful our thoughts can be.

During a pain episode or experience, the more you use catastrophic thinking, the more pain you will have. Thoughts heighten your response to pain. Even when you have a causal reason for the pain—such as I did with my bulging disc—your thought process is important to turning up or down the volume on pain.

Catastrophic thoughts can take various forms. They can be based on anxiety over the pain and worry about the future. Negative thinking is often involved when something we value, like our functioning, is threatened or can be lost or diminished. Fear can prompt this thinking, especially when it is related to our health. Catastrophic thoughts can also be generated in the mind when a situation is vague or ambiguous. In those instances, we tend to fill in the blanks with worst-case scenarios because we don't know outcomes or reasons for our pain.

When catastrophic thinking takes hold, it can impact our relationships. Such thoughts may lead us to socially communicate our distress. The more we complain, the more we hope those around us will react with help. This may be a way of coping and getting others involved in our need for help. But when this happens, research reveals that we may receive critical responses from partners.[3] Thus, the support that is desired may actually put a strain on relationships. The longer the pain persists, the more likely the interpersonal strain. The partner with chronic pain is often viewed as dependent and constantly needing support—another reason to stop this type of thinking.

Another problem is that when catastrophic thinking finds a highway in the brain, it can lead to depression, anxiety, and hopelessness. It can be difficult to focus away from the pain when we perceive the pain as unusually intense and feel helpless to do anything about it. And catastrophic thinking can alter pain. It can actually facilitate the pathway to pain.[4]

Identifying and Changing Catastrophic Thoughts

There is a thirteen-item self-reporting pain scale you can use to see how much you think in catastrophic ways. The pain scale is called the Pain Catastrophizing Scale and was developed by a group of researchers to better understand the pain experience.[5] It helps you rate the frequency of your pain-related thoughts and see how much you ruminate on, magnify, and feel helpless about your pain. You think of a pain experience and then answer the questions. Once you identify your thoughts, you can work to change those thoughts.

Catastrophic thinking gains ground in three ways. First, you ruminate on a thought: *Hmm, I wonder if something bad might happen to me.* Second, you magnify that thought: *I can't seem to get this pain to go away.* Third, you think you are helpless: *I can't go on like this. I can't take it anymore. There is nothing I can do to make it stop.* You have pain, but instead of staying calm and waiting to see if it wanes, you begin to think the worst: *Oh no, not again. This is my life.* This creates stress and anxiety and becomes a thought habit. When this type of appraisal is made, you react in ways that don't help the pain process.

How do you change this? You begin by adjusting your perspective. You can't always avoid pain, but you can adjust your thoughts about the experience. Just because you have pain today doesn't mean you will have pain tomorrow. The key is to stop the distortions and become more reasonable. For example, when I would begin to think, *I will never ice-skate again and will have to live with this pain for the rest of my life,* it simply wasn't true. The recovery process was difficult, but I am able to skate again (I'll forgo the flying camels!) and don't have the pain any longer.

In order to change your thinking, you have to practice removing old thought patterns. First, you identify the catastrophic thought. Thoughts are often automatic, and you may not realize you have such negative thoughts. So recognizing your self-talk is a starting point. Second, you tell yourself to stop and examine the evidence for that thought. Finally, you replace that thought with something less distorted. Start small. Take one thought captive. Confine it and replace it. This process is a way to take responsibility for the management of your pain. Doing so will help you feel a sense of mastery over the parts of the pain experience you can control.

Now there may be some truth in a catastrophic thought. You have to examine the validity of what you are thinking and challenge the aspects of the thought that might be untrue. If you don't, your thoughts can be a self-fulfilling prophecy and lead to the outcome you fear. A self-perpetuating cycle ensues, stress hormones are spiked, and your reactions are out of sync with reality.

The following chart provides an example of how to self-monitor catastrophic thoughts and take them captive. You can use a notebook with four columns to track your own catastrophic thinking.

SITUATION THAT TRIGGERS PAIN	CATASTROPHIC THOUGHT	EVIDENCE FOR THE THOUGHT	REPLACEMENT THOUGHT
Inability to throw a ball	My pain is awful, and there is nothing I can do about it.	I tried only once and couldn't do it. I have thrown a soft Nerf ball in the house. I have days when it doesn't hurt so much.	I have good and bad days. I will throw the ball around on a good day.
Time to get out of bed	It hurts too much. I must be really sick. Something is terribly wrong.	There are days I have gotten out of bed.	I can make my-self get up and out of bed.

Situation that triggers pain: In this column, write down the situations that trigger your pain experiences (when you move about, deal with stress, have marital problems, are more physical, and so on). When you feel pain and begin to think about the negative consequences associated with it, notice what was happening or what you were doing before the pain hit.

Catastrophic thought: What are you thinking when the pain comes? Be mindful of the thoughts that run through your head. Recognize the irrational or catastrophizing thoughts. These types of thoughts go beyond *I am hurting today* to *Hurting means I will never get better*. Once you identify the extreme thought, you can change it. Take the thought captive. Confine it. Say, "Stop!" Sometimes we think our thoughts are rational until we see them on paper. Remember also that your thoughts can be unconscious and automatic, so you have to bring them to your awareness. It may take a new focus to learn to recognize your thoughts. Notice when you use words such as *should, ought, must, never,* and *always.* These words usually signal a thought distortion.

Evidence for the thought: What supports this thought? What works against it? Are there times it isn't true? Does the thought come when you feel something negative like anger, sadness, or anxiety? Would you say this thought out loud to someone? Are there other explanations? Is the bad thing happening now? The threat of pain or the experience of it could be causing you to discount the evidence and overestimate the probability of pain. So ask, *Does the evidence support my pain story?*

Replacement thought: After you have identified the catastrophic thought and looked for evidence to support it (and found none!), replace it with a more tempered or rational thought. The best approach is to put a positive thought in place: *I had one good day; I can have others.* The more positive, the less catastrophizing, the less pain. Consider the positive, more rational thought and believe your thoughts are making a difference.

Once you track your thinking, you must practice *changing* your thinking in order for your brain to use new highways. It is okay to acknowledge that bad things happen. Life is filled with unpleasant moments, seasons, and trials. An acceptance of this basic belief helps when it is accompanied by the understanding that you *do* have control over your *reactions* to difficult events. As a person thinks, so he or she shall be!

The body, the brain, and the mind communicate with one another and are part of the pain process. Thoughts create a reaction in which the brain releases neurotransmitters, those chemical messengers that allow the brain to communicate with parts of itself and the nervous system. The thoughts that flow through the mind sculpt the brain, firing neurons in distinctive ways, forming patterns. Thoughts literally program the cells to receive negative or positive messages. Perceptions, attitudes, and thoughts are involved in controlling biology.

Positive mental self-care directly impacts your physical health. Thus, creating the positive mind-set discussed earlier is important when dealing with pain. Thoughts are so powerful that even the anticipation of pain can trigger pain. Change your thoughts, change your pain.

14

Change Your Emotions, Change Your Pain

If you want to conquer fear, don't sit at home and think about it. Go out and get busy.

Dale Carnegie

Physical pain can often cause anxiety, fear, anger, depression, a sense of helplessness, frustration, guilt, and shame. The more chronic pain becomes, the more emotions can play a role. And emotions can change how we perceive pain. Because the mind and the body are so connected, negative emotions can make chronic pain worse. If you want to live beyond pain, pay attention to how you feel. Controlling your feelings can help you manage pain.[1]

Emotional health is critical to our well-being and self-care. A goal of pain management is to reduce the occurrence of negative emotions and increase the occurrence of positive ones. Paying attention to emotions is one way to turn down the volume on pain. After you understand more about the important connection between pain and emotions, you can apply strategies aimed at improving your emotional health.

Emotions and the Brain

Emotions and chronic pain are interconnected in the brain. Nerves fire and chemicals are secreted in complex physical interactions. Neurotransmitters send information about pain and emotions between nerves. The area of the brain that forms and registers emotions surrounds the pain-processing center, and both these centers activate the same regions of the brain and carry the same neural signatures. Basically, pain and emotions share brain real estate. This is why pain is both a physical and an emotional experience.

Remember that pain is processed in the brain, so what you feel and how you interpret it will establish patterns in the brain. Those patterns influence your present moment and mood, and if emotional patterns are negative, you could have more pain.

To better understand how the brain and emotions work together, let's take a closer look at the central nervous system, specifically the brain. It is made up of two types of tissue: white matter and gray matter. Gray matter is involved in processing information in the brain. It includes multiple regions of the brain that involve sensory perception, speech, memory, decision-making, self-control, muscle control, and emotions. White matter is more like the subway of the brain, transporting functional information and connecting different regions of gray matter to one another. With chronic pain, gray matter can experience a reduction in volume.[2] This happens naturally as a person ages, but it also happens with chronic pain.[3] A reduced volume of gray matter is associated with how our senses and emotions process pain. Chronic pain structurally changes the brain—making pain worse. While we don't quite understand all the changes in brain structures, we do believe that this reduction of gray matter due to chronic pain is likely reversible with treatment.[4] Treatment that includes a focus on changing negative thoughts and emotions helps the brain structurally.[5]

When your emotions have trouble quieting down, it is like your brain is stuck in full throttle. What develops is a hypervigilance to pain and pain-related information. And if you anticipate that a painful experience could result, you want to avoid it.

Since what we emotionally feel influences how we physically feel, negative emotions, like anger, sadness, and depression, can fuel pain. And pain can fuel those emotions. It works both ways. So assessing and working on your emotional well-being is one way to help with chronic pain. As we learn more about this intimate connection between emotions and pain, remember that our discussion is not meant to blame you but rather to empower you to take charge of your emotions and develop a positive mind-set. Change your feelings, change your brain—and change your pain.

Fear and Pain

One of the problems with chronic pain is the anticipation of it. Anticipation is based on prior knowledge and current information regarding something upcoming. Regarding pain, you remember situations and experiences that caused it. As a result, you can become fearful of those experiences and develop anxiety around them. This type of anticipation leads to what is called a fear-avoidance response to chronic pain.

Here is an example to help you think about this in another way. Driving a car is a neutral experience for most of us. But if you are in a car accident, you may develop a fear of driving and avoid it. Now think of this with regard to chronic pain. If you are a back-pain patient and have pain when lifting something, you might become fearful of lifting and avoid lifting all together. Or maybe your doctor told you that lifting heavy objects could result in nerve damage. Or you saw someone lift a heavy object and get hurt. Lifting an object becomes a trigger for expecting pain. You anticipate pain just at the thought of lifting something. Then fear becomes associated with lifting, and you avoid it. Your brain says, "Avoid lifting or there will be pain and possible reinjury." So you become more avoidant and less active, worsening the pain and possibly leading to disability. And fear signals the brain to be hypervigilant and to pay attention to possible threats to your well-being.[6] Once this fear-avoidance is established, it takes work to get rid of it. But you can unlearn this fear and avoidance. Reducing fear-avoidance that develops with chronic pain will help your pain.

Fear also creates anxiety. Fear stimulates the thinking that any ache or pain could be problematic, and thus you become anxious. Anxiety is a result of worry about pain causing something to happen. Both anxiety and worry are future oriented. *What if I hurt myself again? What if I make things worse? What if I become even more disabled?* "What if" is based in doubt about the future. Anxiety and worry make you defensive and paralyze forward movement.

Thus, dialing back on fear is important to living beyond pain. Remember that there are things you can do to better control your pain. Pain is not in control of you if you don't allow it to be. Fear can be controlled and calmed down and not allowed to run your emotions.

Since fear can become such a part of the chronic pain process, let's look at how fear heightens pain. Fear is a normal response to an immediate threat. Fear, like pain, is protective: it warns us of danger. Fear is a process in the brain that is like a chain reaction. If your brain detects a threat, it tells your hypothalamus to alert your adrenal glands to rush blood to your muscles. Your physical body begins to prepare to guard against the fear. The emotional center of your brain tells the thinking part to engage. The thinking part then alerts memory, and memory decides if this current threat is life threatening or not. If your brain says you should be afraid, your brain remembers this and tells you to avoid in the future whatever is happening in that moment. That threat is then hard to forget. The fear pathway that develops can be ramped up over and over and cause you to react quickly to fear. Learned fear can basically trick your memory and perception of reality. Your current situation looks scary, and your brain confirms this.

If you believe pain is a signal that something is terribly wrong, you won't forget it. Then if you react to pain with immense fear, thinking it is dangerous or terrible, you set off the fear response that amps up pain. When that happens, you want to get out of the pain, so you avoid what caused it or reach for a painkiller rather than learn to tolerate the pain. Over time, this avoidance creates more fear and keeps the chronic pain cycle going. While fear is not the source of pain, it can make pain worse. Over time, long-term fear can damage parts of the brain and make regulating it more difficult. This is why we need to calm down fear. The good news is that fear memories can be unlearned.

Fear and anticipation of pain explain why some people experience more pain than others. In fact, researchers found an association between fear levels and impaired functioning of the prefrontal regions of the brain.[7] They noticed a heightened sensitivity to conditioned fear and anxiety-provoking stimuli related to negative emotional regulation. Take away fear and anxiety, and chronic pain lessens. Control fear, and you can better control pain.

While you don't need to understand all the ins and outs of brain science, you should know that regions in the brain associated with processing memory and fear also connect with brain regions associated with pain. What you want to do is create a new response to fear memories and thoughts. You want the thinking part of your brain to reassure the emotional part that you are okay. Your thoughts may not be based on a real threat but on one that has been conditioned in your mind. Emotions follow perceptions.

A key to combating fear is acknowledging that pain—even intense pain at times—is part of life. Accepting this will help moderate your responses to pain and lead to less catastrophic thinking. Pain happens! We don't enjoy it, but we don't have to fear it.

Then you can work to change your perception of fear. The first step is to name the fear. What are you afraid of and why? Be specific. Are you afraid of becoming disabled? Not being able to work? Being dependent on others? If fear is swimming in your brain, name it.

After you name the fear, calm your body down with deep, slow breathing. This decreases tension and stops the feeling of fear from overtaking you. The more you calm down your physical body, the better you can think.

Fear is typically prompted by thoughts of uncertainty, so evaluate your thoughts. Is your fear due to imminent danger, or are you reacting to something imagined? If your fear is based on anxious thinking such as *What if . . .* , then refocus your thoughts to something more positive and hopeful. Tell yourself something like, "I can handle this. I know I can react differently. This pain is difficult, but I can live through it and do things to help myself." This will change your thoughts associated with that fear memory. The more you expose yourself to the fear and know you can work your way through it or handle it, the less power it will have.

In addition to these steps, we encourage you to pay attention to the spiritual part of your life when dealing with chronic pain and fear. You are body, mind, and spirit—all parts influence your daily life. While fear is often based in uncertainty, faith can empower you to trust God for help. In the Old Testament of the Bible, the prophet Isaiah reminds us of a promise from God: "Even to your old age and gray hairs I am he, I am he who will sustain you. I have made you and I will carry you; I will sustain you and I will rescue you" (Isa. 46:4). Fear is a battle that can be fought on the faith front.

If you have a faith perspective, present your fear to God. Ask him to take that fear and fill you with his love. Love overcomes fear. When you know someone loves you and has your back, you can calm down and trust. Know that God will walk with you through this difficult time of pain.

Here is an example of faith in action to conquer fear. When David was up against a powerful Philistine army, he was afraid. He had just escaped a terrifying incident in the middle of enemy territory and wrote these words recorded in Psalms: "I sought the LORD, and he answered me; he delivered me from all my fears" (34:4). It is possible to be delivered from fear and to have peace in the middle of pain when faith is employed.

Faith helps us focus on the positives of the future. Faith reminds us that we will get through our present situations. In times of fear, remind yourself of this. You will get through it. So battle against fear with your mind and spirit. War against unbelief that tells you there is no help or hope. Hold up a shield of faith against the arrows of fear. Face your fear, name it, change your negative thought to a positive, and fear has to leave.

In sum, fear can come from traumatic experiences such as an accident or an injury, but avoiding fear allows it to grow. Pain-related fear creates avoidance that can lead to disability. Fear can be more disabling than the original injury because fear keeps avoidance going. Fear can cause you to interpret any pain as catastrophic. Fear can lead to being hypervigilant about pain, which means you are on high alert and attending to it. Fear can stop you from doing things that gradually you could do. Fear can lead to depression and anxiety. Basically, fear can stop you from accomplishing your goals and purpose in life. You don't have to live in fear. You can be empowered to face it and overcome it.

Anger and Pain

Pamela experienced diffuse pain every day. When she woke up, she had pain in her muscles and joints, in her neck and back—all over. It persisted all day. She lost sleep. She struggled at home and at work.

Pamela's pain began two years earlier with no apparent physical cause or injury. Numerous doctors' visits and tests yielded no diagnosis. Frustratingly, Pamela was stuck with this unexplained pain. However, a therapist talked to her about an emotional trauma she had endured years ago and wondered if the trauma could be related to her pain. Pamela didn't recognize the link between the pain and her emotions until she was brought to a place of desperation.

Pamela had endured the death of her thirty-four-year-old son, who, while driving his motorcycle, had been struck by another driver. It is difficult to describe the emotional pain that occurs when a parent loses a child, especially when it occurs in an accident that, on all accounts, shouldn't have happened. Pamela was riddled with sadness, but she was also angry. The other driver was responsible for the accident, and she wanted him to pay. She wanted him to lose sleep at night. She wanted him to experience loss. She wanted him to feel the pain that she was suffering.

One day Pamela was driving on the highway and sensed that it was time to let go of her anger and forgive this man or she would never move forward in her life. Her anger was becoming her focus in life. She pulled her car off the road and surrendered the anger, the disgust, and the sense of injustice. Something happened in that moment. In her heart, she released the man she felt was responsible, but she was the one set free. From that moment, she had peace. Later, when people would ask how she was doing or about her son, the anger that once had boiled beneath the surface wasn't there. She was beginning to heal.

Then Pamela had a realization. Not long after that moment of releasing her anger, she noticed that she was not having as much pain, and over time, her pain was almost gone. Though the sorrow from losing her son would never fully go away, the pain that resulted from that loss no longer ruled her life.

In life, all of us suffer loss and sometimes experience tragedy. It is normal to experience sorrow and anger in response to life's difficult times. But Pamela's story demonstrates the power of negative emotions, particularly anger, and how it can influence our physiology because we are integrated beings. We cannot separate what happens in the mind from what happens in the body. While your pain may not be rooted in anger, take inventory to see if anger could be increasing your pain.

When loss is a part of life, even when the loss is associated with chronic pain, you go through stages of grief. At first, there is denial: "I can't have my life changed like this." At times, there is pleading and bargaining: "Please, God, take this pain away. I just want to feel normal." Feelings of sadness, depression, and anxiety come and go. And so do feelings of anger, especially when you realize that there isn't a quick fix or chronic pain may linger. Whatever the cause, acknowledge anger as part of the normal process of dealing with pain. Feel it, but don't hang on to it. If you do, it could become resentment and even bitterness. Here are some suggestions to help you move through the normal phase of anger that comes with chronic pain.

Admit you are angry. When you repress anger, you feel anger but do not acknowledge or express it. You feel it but deny it. You may have learned this growing up. Maybe you were told not to get angry. Maybe your parents repressed their anger because they didn't want you to be afraid. Maybe you've had bad experiences with anger and feeling out of control.

Denying or repressing the emotion can lead to overeating, boredom, depression, anxiety, physical illness, gossip, and so on. Repressed anger can build up and lead to resentment. Theodore Rubin, a New York psychoanalyst, believes repressed anger is the source of much anxiety. In his book *The Angry Book*, he talks about repressed anger as a major root of anxiety disorders.[8] Repressing anger can be a temporary solution to not dealing with an issue but one that causes physical and emotional problems. When you are angry, identify the feeling and decide to work through it. Talking to someone may help.

Identify the source of your anger. What makes you mad? Usually this is based on thoughts of injustice. Pain isn't fair. Other times anger may be directed at family members who seem insensitive, doctors who don't give you what you need, and people who are healthy. Recognize the things that set you off so you can be intentional concerning your reaction.

Don't make excuses for your anger. For example, "I'm in pain, so, yes, I can lose my temper." "My wife makes me so mad because she doesn't understand what I'm going through." Be angry, but don't go after someone because you are in pain. Anger is normal, but the way you behave when angry can be healthy or unhealthy. Exercise control when dealing with feelings of anger.

Don't jump to conclusions. Is your anger based on a real situation, or is it based on your perception? Sometimes we misread people and believe they have hurt us when they haven't. For example, you might get angry because your partner hasn't been talking much and you think it is because they don't care about you or the pain you're in. But it may be that your partner is going through a rough time at work and didn't want to tell you because they didn't want to upset you and make your pain worse, not because they don't care. Our misreading of a problem can lead to anger, making our pain worse. We can easily become the victim. Therefore, take time to clarify the situation that made you angry and get more facts.

Refuse to keep thinking about the injustice that is fueling your anger. Once you have identified the source of your anger, let it go and begin to move toward acceptance. This is a process and may involve confronting your anger about being in pain all the time. It isn't fair to be in pain but it is reality. So rather than getting stuck on the injustice, accept the reality of life being unfair at times and learn to cope by controlling the part you can—your reaction to the pain.

Don't vent. When you express anger by screaming, yelling, punching pillows, and so on, you actually increase anger instead of reduce it. Venting does not make anger go away but revs it up.

Practice self-soothing and calming methods. This book contains many ways to calm yourself down. They are directed at engaging the rational versus the emotional part of your brain. Count to ten before acting. Take slow, deep breaths. Use distraction and stress management (discussed later).

Be assertive and confrontational, not aggressive. When you become angry at anyone or anything, keep your pain levels down by learning to be assertive not aggressive. Learn to confront people and problems in a well-controlled manner that won't lead to aggression and more anger.

Holding on to anger disrupts feelings of well-being. It impacts physical health. In fact, repressed anger activates stress hormones and makes us more prone to illness.[9] We always have a choice. How we deal with anger is in our control. Don't repress it and hope it doesn't affect you. Instead, deal with the issue and let it go.

Depression and Pain

Depression is common among people with chronic pain.[10] If you are constantly stressed, angry, or anxious due to pain, it can be depressing. Pain lowers your frustration threshold and impacts your sleep, exercise, relationships, work, and social life. It can lead to feelings of helplessness and powerlessness because of the losses felt.

Doctors have known for a long time that pain and depression are linked. They share the same brain messengers that travel between nerves and travel on the same highways in the brain and spinal cord. This is one reason why certain antidepressants help reduce the perception of pain—they involve the same nerves and neurotransmitters.

Depression can make pain worse, and chronic pain can bring on depression.[11] The more depressed you are, the harder pain is to tolerate. Remember, your nervous system is stuck in that high-reactivity pattern, meaning your threshold for pain is lowered. Depression can influence the intensity, frequency, and healing of your pain. At times, depression can cause unexplained physical symptoms of pain. And sometimes symptoms such as chronic joint pain, limb pain, gastrointestinal problems, tiredness, sleep problems, and so on can be indicators of depression.[12] In fact, if you present with a high number of physical symptoms, you are more likely to have a mood disorder than someone who has only a few physical complaints.[13] And the more painful those physical symptoms, the more severe the depression can be. Physical symptoms can also increase the duration of depression.[14]

Depression can lead to suicidal thoughts and even attempts. According to University of Miami professor David Fishbain, this is not uncommon among chronic pain patients. Chronic pain is considered a suicide risk factor.[15] Therefore, if you are depressed, get treatment for both the depression and the physical symptoms. If you don't, there is a higher chance of relapse.[16] You need both the depression and the pain to be in remission in order to live beyond pain.

When pain and depression coexist, the combination often goes undiagnosed. Early diagnosis is key. If you experience signs of anxiety, persistent sadness, difficulty falling or staying asleep, feelings of hopelessness, loss of pleasure doing things that used to bring pleasure, concentration problems, an increase or decrease in appetite, low energy, lack of motivation, feelings of worthlessness, psychomotor agitation or restlessness, and suicidal thoughts, you may be depressed. If these symptoms sound and feel familiar, see a mental health professional to be evaluated. Depression is generally treatable, and treatment will improve your pain.

Antidepressants and Pain

As noted earlier, there is evidence that antidepressant medication can be helpful to some people with chronic pain, particularly when used to treat neuropathic pain such as diabetic neuropathy and post-herpetic neuralgia.[17] One thought is that antidepressants increase neurotransmitters in the spinal cord that might reduce pain signals and impact at the cerebral level as well.[18] And both chronic pain syndromes and depression involve inflammation, a common denominator that can be helped with antidepressants.[19] Since chronic pain and depression share neurobiology and neuro-anatomy, whether you are depressed or not, these medications may help.[20] But remember, antidepressants don't work immediately, so it may take a few weeks for you to feel some relief.

If you recall from a previous chapter, the types of antidepressants often used are the older versions called tricyclics, which do have several side effects. Doses are typically low and started slowly in order to reduce some of these side effects. The newer versions of antidepressants called serotonin and norepinephrine reuptake inhibitors (SNRIs) are also frequently used in chronic pain treatment and have fewer side effects. Another class of antidepressants that has fewer side effects is selective serotonin reuptake inhibitors (SSRIs). These can increase suicidal thoughts in some people, so they need to be administered and managed by a physician.

You don't have to be depressed to benefit from antidepressants when chronic pain is involved.[21] The FDA has approved many anti-depressants for use with various chronic pain conditions.[22] So talk to your doctor as to whether or not antidepressants should be part of your treatment. In order to decide if medication is a treatment option you want to pursue, you will need to review your medication history and weigh the benefits and cost of using antidepressants with your physician. Side effects can be significant and need to be discussed.

Here's the takeaway on emotions and pain: there is a strong connection between them. Negative emotions such as fear, anger, and depression all turn up the volume on pain. But those emotions can be regulated and managed, making your emotional life a source of pain management.

15

Change Your Relationships, Change Your Pain

> When we honestly ask ourselves which person in our lives means the most to us, we often find that it is those who, instead of giving advice, solutions, or cures, have chosen rather to share our pain and touch our wounds with a warm and tender hand.
>
> Henri Nouwen

Perhaps one of the most overlooked areas in treating chronic pain is the way it impacts relationships. Our relationships are important in our daily lives and greatly influence our mood and functioning. Pain affects relationships, and relationships affect people in pain. So it makes sense to pay attention to this critical part of our lives. Relationships can contribute to pain or help a person deal with it.

Family

Living with someone in chronic pain can be demanding at times and bring up feelings of powerlessness because you can't make their pain stop. But people in pain need emotional support. There is, however, a fine line between helping and hurting when it comes to chronic pain. If you are in a relationship with a person in chronic pain, you want to give the right kind of support.

If you are overprotective with a person in pain, meaning you do everything for them (e.g., get their medications, tell them to rest, take over their responsibilities, etc.), you may be preventing them from getting better. In your zeal to help, you really aren't helping. Doing too much for the person in pain will make them less active, maybe even depressed. It will wear on their sense of independence and reinforce helplessness.

On the other hand, you have to be careful not to be punitive or negative when responding to pain complaints. Statements such as "I don't want to hear about this again" or "It's depressing hearing about your pain all the time" are not helpful either. With couples, punitive statements can erode marital satisfaction.[1]

Toby Newton-John, a clinical psychologist at the University of Technology in Sydney, Australia, studies the social dynamics surrounding chronic pain.[2] He has discovered that the way couples interact around pain matters. The more the focus is on pain and the more a partner does things for the person in pain, the more likely they are to increase the person's disability.

Something as simple as the way a person in pain talks to others can also make a difference in their pain level. Constant conversations about pain will increase pain. So instead of saying, "How are your headaches today?" say, "How is it going today?" This is a subtle but important difference. Instead of focusing on the pain, you are focusing on the person. Here is another example. Instead of saying, "Is your pain worse today?" ask, "Are you feeling yourself today?" The person in pain needs this type of support and empathy.

Children are also affected by a parent in chronic pain. They may feel anxious and not understand why Mom or Dad is in pain. They might respond with anger because a parent isn't participating in activities or family events. Or they may feel guilty, thinking they are doing things to cause the pain or make it worse.

Family roles change because the person in pain isn't functioning like they used to. Others have to step in and pick up the slack. Chronic pain can also be costly, resulting in medical bills that can strain family finances. Family members might feel resentful to have added responsibility. And the person in pain may feel like a burden to those in the family. All of this can add up to relationship tension and frustration. This is why families should be a part of pain treatment. The entire family needs to be educated about chronic pain and how to respond and reorganize in ways that lower tension.

The person in pain must communicate needs directly in order to avoid the buildup of anger and resentment. A pattern of resentment, aversion, and unmet expectations will develop if family members aren't talking and on the same page regarding attitudes and expectations about pain. For instance, what are the expectations when it comes to movement, exercise, help with household tasks, and so on? Pain has changed family life and needs to be acknowledged with realistic goals for reorganizing the family unit. Here is an example.

Bonnie was dealing with fibromyalgia and was married to Tom. Bonnie lost her job due to too many absences, and Tom was feeling the financial strain. Bonnie was also engaging in catastrophic talk. The couple was growing apart, and anger and resentment were building.

Bonnie expected Tom to provide her support but wasn't asking for it directly or being specific about her needs. Instead, she moaned and grimaced, leaving Tom to feel helpless as to what to do. Bonnie felt disappointed not getting what she considered needed support, and Tom had no idea what she expected. Tom was beginning to doubt the reality of Bonnie's pain and didn't understand how Bonnie could be so limited in helping with tasks she'd previously handled. There was a growing emotional distance, a precursor for divorce.

The couple had never worked together on dealing with chronic pain, so when they agreed to therapy, the first step was education about fibromyalgia. Tom attended Bonnie's doctor visits and learned more about the condition. He was able to ask the doctor about expectations regarding Bonnie's movement and participation in physical activities. He and Bonnie learned that moderate activity could help alleviate some of her pain.

One of the issues was that Bonnie did not acknowledge her limits and Tom didn't recognize them. Once they discussed these limits and how they could accommodate them without causing resentment, the couple began to do better. Bonnie admitted that she had become passive about her pain and was expecting Tom to do more for her. Rather than groaning and moaning, she needed to ask for emotional support when she was feeling discouraged. Tom understood that his role was to be a listening ear, not to always try to fix things or do things for Bonnie. Tom also wanted Bonnie to listen to him when he felt helpless regarding her pain. This improved communication helped tremendously.

Bonnie was able to take a job that allowed her to work at home at her own pace. This relieved the financial stress immediately and opened the door to even more conversation. Working through realistic expectations brought Bonnie and Tom closer. Once they learned to communicate and work together, they decided to stay together. They loved each other and needed a better way to keep that love alive. Interestingly, researchers have found that being in love relieves pain.[3] While we can't give a prescription for love, working to restore a loving relationship will help any couple cope better with pain.

Rejection and Isolation

Pain can put you in a bad mood, making you more irritable and less tolerant of others. If you are living with someone who has a job and pain has robbed you of work, you may feel envious and angry. If you can't do your normal part in the household, you may feel like a burden. Maybe you stopped doing the fun physical things you used to do with your family because the pain was too much. You find yourself fixated on your pain, and your world is becoming smaller and smaller. As a result, you may feel isolated. Your marriage may suffer, and friends might disappear.

People in chronic pain often withdraw from family and friends. They hate what pain is doing to their body and feel burdensome to others. Pain often makes them unreliable when it comes to showing up for events or engaging in activities. As a result, they can be rejected.

No one likes to be rejected. It can be devastating and affect how you feel and think about yourself. Stanford researchers found that rejection is so powerful for some people that it can linger for years and cause future problems.[4] This is especially true with romantic rejection. When someone decides they don't care about you or don't want to be with you anymore, it can leave you questioning who you are and what the future might be. But if you have that growth mind-set we discussed earlier, you can grow, develop, bounce back from rejection, and reverse the negativity.

Feeling disconnected from others or being socially excluded by others is actually a risk factor for pain. So bullying, isolation, social rejection, separation, and a lack of support can lead to the body being more sensitized to pain.[5] When this happens, thoughts and emotions are affected and can turn up the volume on pain. Pain can be reinforced.

As we discussed, pain can cause anger. If you are angry and blow up at people, you will alienate them, causing isolation. Stuffing down your anger doesn't solve anything either. Anger, if not dealt with properly, can lead to more rejection and isolation.

Friendships

Friendships are also affected by chronic pain. Friends often have to deal with canceled plans when the person in pain is having a bad day. A cancellation is not personal, but it can feel that way to a friend. So conversations about reliability need to be a part of ongoing friendships. One strategy is to make compromises. If you are dealing with pain, decide that when it becomes difficult, your friend can come to your house rather than meeting at a restaurant, or you can pick a less physical activity for a night out.

Make an effort to do as much as you can to stay connected. Those who love and care about you will appreciate your efforts. The reality is that you will have good days and bad days. When a bad day happens, friends need to remember that despite your lack of participation that day, your good friendship qualities didn't vanish.

A few tips for people who have friends in pain include these:

- Even though the person in pain may cancel on you, continue to include them and invite them to activities so they don't feel left out. If they do cancel because they are having a bad pain day, don't take it personally.

- Encourage rather than criticize. Don't make suggestions as to what they should do unless they ask you. Usually, the friend in pain is doing the best they can and needs to be encouraged to advocate for themselves. If your friend in pain has specific dietary choices that help pain, support those choices. Offer specific help when needed. For example, "I'm running errands tomorrow. Is there something I can pick up for you when I am out?"

- Don't tell a friend that their pain is in their head or could be worse. Also, don't offer platitudes such as "God never gives us more than we can handle" or "Everything happens for a reason." These only make people feel worse. While those statements may be true, they are not comforting in the middle of a pain episode.

- Be flexible. Plans will change. Let the person in pain set the pace. Flexibility is a practical way to support someone in pain.

- Be present. Good friends stick together through good and bad times. Assure your friend that you will be there to support them. People with chronic pain will tell you that your support is a gift. The fact that you understand is powerful.

A patient with cancer pain once said to me (Linda) that having pain and cancer didn't mean she was not a person. She knew that her pain meant she wasn't always fun and had some really bad days, but she needed friends to love and support her. Sometimes she couldn't do things because of the pain, but other times she could, so she wanted friends to keep asking her to do things to bring normalcy to her life. Most important was that she needed people to listen to her, as her journey with pain and cancer was rough and she didn't want to go it alone. Her message: keep reaching out, keep checking in, keep people in your prayers.

The best thing friends can do is provide empathy and keep checking in with those living with chronic pain. When people feel listened to and validated, they have less pain.[6] In fact, most of us do better in life when we feel heard and understood.

Sex and Intimacy

When you are in chronic pain, the last thing you may be thinking about is sex. With chronic pain, you hurt or may lack sexual desire due to the pain and medications taken. For example, sexual dysfunction is a common side effect of chronic opioid use.[7] Yet sexual function is an important part of intimate relationships.

Intimate relationships can be challenged depending on the intensity and source of pain. It may take more talking and intention to keep an active sex life alive. You may have to experiment and try new positions for sexual encounters or use lubrication and other aids to make sex more enjoyable. Ways to increase touch and stimulation are important to discuss as well.

Talk about what feels good and what causes pain. Have a goal to stay connected sexually, as this is a way to increase the body's natural painkillers, endorphins. They are released through touch and sexual encounters. It may also help to limit alcohol and tobacco use, as these can impair sexual function as well. Find ways to relax, enjoy each other, and laugh. Stay positive during setbacks. Talk through intimacy problems when they arise in order to maintain an emotional connection. The more intimate you are with those you love, the better your coping will be.

Intimacy is more than a physical act. It includes talking, touching, and caring as well as sex. Intimate conversations may include your worry about rejection, performance, and whether your partner is finding you less interested or less attractive due to the effects of pain. All of these are good areas to discuss and are part of the process of building intimacy.

Building nonsexual ways to be intimate is also important. Develop common interests that you can do together. Plan for the time of day or night when you have the most energy. Get rest. Spend time together and build your friendship as a foundation for an intimate relationship.

Relationships are important to people in pain, though they shouldn't revolve around pain. If you are in a relationship with someone in pain, be a good listener and encourage as much independence as possible. If you are the person dealing with pain, do not isolate yourself; work to keep relationships strong. The more you and your family can discuss and be educated about the consequences of pain, the stronger your family unit can be and the more you can help one another cope with life's challenges.

16

Change Your Stress, Change Your Pain

If you don't think your anxiety, depression, sadness and stress impact your physical health, think again. All of these emotions trigger chemical reactions in your body, which can lead to inflammation and a weakened immune system. Learn how to cope, sweet friend. There will always be dark days.

Kris Carr

As discussed in chapter 8, stress can make you more vulnerable to pain and make pain worse. To help manage the effects of stress, your muscles need to relax, your breathing needs to slow down, and your mind needs to be at peace and focused in more positive ways.

Stress can be reduced in several ways. The following are a few methods that have been shown to help people with chronic pain. If one or two of these methods seem to resonate with you, practice them for a few weeks. See if they reduce your pain. There is no one way to manage stress, but if you can change your stress, you can change your pain.

Distraction

When you are in pain, several areas of the brain are at work. If you can distract your brain from the pain and focus on something new, your pain will decrease. You can do this in several ways:

- Increase touch sensation by rubbing lotion on your skin and attending to the way it feels.
- Hold something in your hand and focus your attention on how it feels.
- Smell something like a candle and focus your attention on the smell.
- Attend to positive sensations in your body, not the pain.
- Move and focus on the movement.
- Create peaceful images in your brain to flood your brain with new senses and thoughts.
- Distract yourself with reading, watching a movie, listening to music, knitting, painting, talking to a friend—anything that pulls your attention off the pain.

Relaxation Methods

Relaxation seems so obvious, yet we often forget these simple methods to relieve stress.

Deep Breathing

Deep breathing is an easy technique that can be used throughout the day. You can use this in bed, sitting in a chair, or in most other situations. It takes only a few minutes and can lower stress, reduce tension, and help you relax, thereby decreasing your pain.

When you become stressed, breathing tends to become shallow and this limits the diaphragm's range of motion. As a result, the lowest parts of your lungs don't receive fully oxygenated air. Deep breathing corrects this as well as slows down your heart rate and stabilizes blood pressure. It also takes your mind off pain by refocusing your thoughts on your breathing.

If you are able (not when you are driving a car), find a comfortable position. Begin to breathe normally. Think of your stomach as a balloon that you want to inflate and deflate through slow and intentional breathing. Unless your eyes need to be open, close your eyes and focus on each breath. Begin by inhaling through your nose and holding your breath for a count of four, then exhale through your mouth or nose for a count of four. Repeat this ten times. If you place your hand on your stomach, you should feel your diaphragm moving in and out. You can check yourself by placing one hand on your stomach and the other on your chest. The hand on your stomach should move, and the hand on your chest should remain still.

If you desire, you can add a short, repetitive prayer or phrase to your deep breathing. A phrase such as "God is good" or "God loves me" can remind you to focus on God's presence along with each breath. Both deep breathing and repetitive prayer help with anxiety as well.

As you concentrate on each breath and intentionally slow down your breathing, your body relaxes. Relaxation helps lessen pain because it is the opposite of tension. Notice how you feel at the end of this type of practice. The more you practice, the easier it will be to use deep breathing when you feel stressed. We like this technique because it is portable and easy to learn and do.

Progressive Muscle Relaxation

Once you master deep breathing, you can combine it with a technique designed to relax your muscles called progressive muscle relaxation.[1] While practicing deep breathing, close your eyes and focus on one part of your body or group of muscles. Tense the muscle group for several seconds, focus on how that tension feels, then relax the muscles and study the difference between tension and relaxation. For example, make a fist and tense the muscles of your arm, study the tension, then relax your arm. Notice the relaxation and how different it feels from tension. You can apply this sequence to all the muscle groups until your entire body is relaxed.

This works best if you can tense and relax muscles without exacerbating your pain. If you encounter pain with tensing, you may want to gently stretch a series of muscles. Once you can stretch the muscles, you can slowly add in progressive muscle relaxation. Again, the more you practice this, the easier it will be to relax your body. There are scripts on the internet that can walk you through the progression of muscle relaxation. You simply download the app or web tool, then listen and follow the instructions to tense and relax. Using this at bedtime also helps with sleep.

Guided Imagery

Guided imagery can work for all kinds of pain, but it is especially helpful for arthritis and other joint diseases in which you are aware of pain in various parts of your body.[2] Guided imagery can be used anywhere. It is a visualization technique validated as a way to reduce stress and pain. It uses your thoughts to distract you from the pain and lower the level of stress hormones. Basically, it calms down the sympathetic nervous system. By employing this technique, you slow down respiration, heart rate, and blood pressure. Chemicals such as serotonin, norepinephrine, and dopamine are released, decreasing stress, pain levels, fear, and anxiety.

To begin, think of a relaxing scene—a place that seems peaceful and calming. Choose a setting that is personally soothing or is based on a positive memory. It might be a quiet cabin in the woods, a beach in the Caribbean, or a snowy mountain ski lodge. Next, develop that scene in great detail in your mind using all your senses. Imagine the colors, sounds, smells. Complete the scene and then visualize yourself in that scene. Immerse yourself in it. Take a deep breath and visualize the scene playing out. Doing this will put you in a state of relaxation and lower anxiety. As a result, your pain will decrease. Here is an example:

> Imagine yourself lying on a beach. The sand is white and warm. Sunlight is dancing on the water. You dig your feet into the sand, feeling the coolness of the layers. You hear the soft crashing of small waves on the shore. A gentle breeze is blowing on your face, providing a slight coolness. You smell the salt from the ocean water and observe the white, fluffy clouds in the sky as a seagull swoops by.

Do this whenever you begin to feel tension in your body. You don't have to spend an hour doing this; rather, when you feel stressed, stop what you are doing, picture yourself in that relaxing place, imagine the scene as vividly as you can, and go there for a moment. Your body will relax.

If you have difficulty fully imagining a scene by yourself, there are prerecorded guided imagery sessions available on the internet that can be downloaded, listened to, or purchased. There are also podcasts that can be downloaded for personal use. However you do it, this practice will improve movement and function. The use of guided imagery has been shown to reduce the need for nonsteroidal anti-inflammatory drugs (NSAIDs) and other pain medications.[3]

Autogenic Training

Related to guided imagery, autogenic training involves autonomic self-regulation. A number of your vital organs depend on basic functions, like breathing and digesting food, that keep the body stable. Your autonomic nervous system is a control system in your body that unconsciously regulates body functions such as heart rate, digestion, and breathing. The idea of this technique is to learn to regulate autonomic sensations by blocking out environmental distractions, focusing on specific imagery, and normalizing the physiological systems.

Basically, the training involves imagining a calm, relaxing environment and focusing on comfortable body sensations—heaviness and warmth in the limbs, cardiac regulation, breathing, warmth in the upper abdomen, and coolness on the forehead. The idea is to change your pain sensations to a more soothing sensation, such as warmth. To do this, you need to learn a series of six formulas related to autonomic sensations. They are

1. a feeling of heaviness related to muscle relaxation;
2. a feeling of warmth in the arms related to vascular dilation;
3. heartbeat related to stabilization of heart function;
4. regulation of breathing;
5. a feeling of warmth in the abdomen related to the regulation of visceral organs;
6. coolness on the forehead related to blood flow in the head.[4]

To practice, find a comfortable position, take a few deep breaths, and say to yourself, "I am completely calm." Then the focus on specific areas of the body begins. For example, say, "My arms are really heavy, warm, and relaxed." Repeat this a few times. Then move to another part of your body, such as your legs, and do the same. Focus your attention on calm and regular breathing. You can say, "My heartbeat is calm and regular" as you progress in the relaxation. Then move to your abdomen and say, "My abdomen is warm, and I am completely calm." Do this a few times and then move to your forehead. "My forehead is cool and relaxed." Repeat this sequence of heavy, warm, and cool.[5]

Usually, an instructor teaches this so you can learn the procedure and do it on your own. Like all relaxation techniques, it has to be practiced over time so you can teach your body to relax and regulate stress. This technique is not recommended for people with heart conditions, those with psychotic symptoms, children below the age of five, or those whose symptoms you can't control during the training.[6]

A Warm Bath

Pain sufferers often use a warm bath as a way to relax. Sitting in a hot tub helps decrease stress hormones and release endorphins, the body's painkillers. Adding a lavender scent to the water aids relaxation as well. As you soak, focus on the aroma of the lavender and the hot, soothing water, and your body will calm down.

Massage

I (Linda) am a big believer in massage, partly because I love the way it makes me feel. There is something so relaxing about lying down on a warm massage table and having someone work through your tense muscles. It relaxes the mind and the body. The downside is that massage can be expensive. However, some massage schools provide inexpensive massages because their students need the practice. Lifestyle centers in hospitals may also provide inexpensive massages. If you can find a good massage therapist, can afford it, and can tolerate the touch, massage can help relieve your stress and reduce your pain.

Biofeedback

Biofeedback is used to treat a number of chronic pain conditions, such as headaches, fibromyalgia, and rheumatoid arthritis.[7] It teaches you how to read physiological feedback from a machine to learn how your body responds and reacts to stress and pain. The goal is to gain voluntary control and to self-regulate specific physiological responses in order to reduce pain.

Biofeedback treatments require the use of a monitoring device designed to measure several physiological processes—heart rate, muscle tension, galvanic skin response (changes in sweat gland activity)—in order for you to learn how to control physiological arousal using your mind. Electric sensors are attached to certain organs or muscle groups, and you use a number of strategies, such as deep breathing, to control your physical body based on the feedback you receive from the machine. Using the device, you are able to bring under control formerly involuntary physical responses. Usually, ten to twenty treatments are required to master the technique.

The training can be done in physical therapy clinics, medical centers, and hospitals. Home devices are available, and apps can also be downloaded that monitor your breathing through a sensor worn on the body. If you are interested in learning biofeedback, consult your physician or mental health professional for places to train. This is a noninvasive way to manage stress and take charge of your health.

Hypnosis

Hypnosis is another technique used to manage the stress related to chronic pain.[8] At the present time, we do not completely understand the neurological mechanisms that cause a state of hypnosis.[9] Imaging studies show changes in the brain in response to hypnotic suggestions but determine only the effects of hypnosis, not the state itself.

Not everyone responds to hypnosis. In fact, only a small percentage of people are believed to be "highly hypnotizable." In fMRIs, people who are susceptible to hypnosis show connections in the brain not seen in those low in hypnotizability.

Hypnosis is a redirection of the brain's attention away from certain thoughts. In a relaxed and comfortable state, critical-thinking skills and decision-making parts of the brain aren't needed. You are absorbed in the moment and not worrying about other things. According to David Spiegel, a Stanford brain researcher who studies fMRIs related to hypnosis, the hypnotic brain doesn't worry about anything, which helps the brain process and control what is going on in the body, and lessens the person's awareness regarding actions. This means that when you are engaged in hypnosis, you don't think about your actions. You just do something based on the power of suggestion.[10] Core beliefs are still present, but during the hypnotic state, the decision-making filter is not as active, allowing the power of suggestion to be implanted. You are open to influence but do not do things against your own will.

Hypnosis can be thought of as a state of selective attention.[11] Heightened attention minimizes distractions and increases responsiveness to suggestions. Pulse and respiration also slow down. Once relaxed, a person receives a suggestion from a hypnotherapist that is specific to the nature of their pain. For example, "Your pain will feel annoying, not excruciating." Basically, a hypnotist focuses the attention of the patient, suggests relaxing the body, gives a suggestion to change the experience of pain, and then debriefs the person with a posthypnotic suggestion.

In my (Linda's) work, patients sometimes raise a concern about the use of hypnosis because it gives power to another person to put suggestions in your mind. The question often asked is whether an altered state of consciousness can open doors in the spiritual realm. Overall, the power of suggestion is not something to be taken lightly, whether it involves hypnosis or conscious words in everyday living. We can be influenced, not controlled, by many things contending for our minds. We are to guard our minds and keep them positive.

Therefore, this technique should be used only with someone you trust and who shares your worldview. If you have concerns about using hypnosis, there are plenty of other tools that can help manage the stress associated with chronic pain.

Mindfulness

Literally hundreds of studies have been published on mindfulness,[12] showing positive changes in the brain. Changes are seen in brain-wiring patterns and in increases in the volume of certain brain regions,[13] resulting in improved well-being. Mindfulness-based therapy approaches such as mindfulness-based stress reduction (MBSR), which you will read about in chapter 19, have been shown to help chronic pain.[14] Mostly, these types of approaches help with symptoms of anxiety and depression. Attending to bodily sensations and mental activities can help one relax and calm down.

Mindfulness, separate from therapy or any spiritual practice, is a technique that helps focus the mind on the present moment. It is about paying attention. It is noticing in the moment what you are thinking, feeling, and doing. It is a nonjudgmental awareness of the present moment. Mindfulness is meant to improve physical and psychological health. It involves a type of acceptance in which you don't judge a feeling or thought but simply acknowledge it exists and accept it.[15] Mindfulness is about being kind to yourself. For most people, it takes about twenty minutes to settle the mind and focus only on the moment because we are easily distracted and future focused.

When mindfulness is taught, you are asked to get in a comfortable position, quiet yourself, and notice your breathing. Breathing is slowed through the use of deep breathing exercises. Then whatever comes into your mind, you observe it and don't try to push it away. Thoughts are like clouds floating through your mind. You allow the thought or emotion to come and go as you focus on the present moment of relaxation.

This approach is widely popular in our culture and has many meanings and uses, as noted by the *New York Times*:

> Mindfulness has come to comprise a dizzying range of meanings for popular audiences. It's an intimately attentive frame of mind. It's a relaxed-alert frame of mind. It's equanimity. It's a form of the rigorous Buddhist meditation called vipassana ("insight"), or a form of another kind of Buddhist meditation known as asanapanasmrti ("awareness of the breath"). It's M.B.S.R. therapy

(mindfulness-based stress reduction). It's just kind of stopping to smell the roses. And last, it's a lifestyle trend, a social movement and—as a *Time* magazine cover had it last year—a revolution.[16]

Mindfulness, although often taught from a Zen Buddhist tradition, does not have to be Buddhist or secular. There are alternative practices of mindfulness that can accommodate other world and faith views. For example, Christianity has a rich tradition of watchfulness. This early Christian term was born out of the ancient practice of contemplative prayer dating back to St. John of the Cross and early contemplatives. Contemplative practices are deeply rooted in Christian orthodoxy. Well-known pastor and author John Piper says, "Contemplation is just another way of talking about spiritually seeing the beauty of Christ in and through the word of God."[17] It is a type of spiritual seeing in which you read the Bible, pause, meditate on it, and allow it to penetrate your soul.

From a Christian perspective, mindfulness is not designed to enhance focused attention on the self or body awareness but on the Trinity. A Trinity focus includes the immanence of God, transcendence, and the reality of God with us. We are never alone as God indwells us.

The tension between secular approaches or Buddhist philosophy and the Christian practice of mindfulness is that the attitudes of acceptance and self-compassion differ. Christianity emphasizes self-awareness related to God as a person. In Buddhist philosophy, there is no God in the Christian sense of a divine being, and there is no sin related to an act of rebellion against God, as noted in original sin. The narratives are different.

So while mindfulness approaches are typically based on Buddhist philosophy and taught in a Westernized way in business and academic settings, the concern for Christians has been the teaching of self-awareness apart from God, the sin nature of humanity, and the indwelling presence of an eternal God as these relate to practice. However, accommodations can be made to incorporate the Christian worldview into the practice. For example, mindfulness for the Christian is not union with the sacred, as some religions espouse. Christians are not one with God nor do they blend themselves into God.

Researcher and professor Fernando Garzon states that the purpose of Christian mindfulness is to deepen one's relationship with God, cultivate spiritual growth and emotional healing, and grow in love toward one another and toward oneself. It includes God, Scripture and self, self-awareness and God-awareness, trust, confession, surrender, and grace.[18] Garzon and Kristy Ford tested a Christian-accommodated form of mindfulness against a traditional form of mindfulness with Christian university students in order to determine if a religiously accommodated form of mindfulness led to better outcomes for Christian students. It did and supported the notion that worldview can be accommodated with this type of technique.[19]

Mindfulness in its essence is learning to control focus and pay attention. Mindfulness is not prayer. Prayer in the Christian tradition is conversation with God. It is not wordless listening. Yes, we listen for a response to our conversations with God, but prayer without words is meditation, not prayer. Mindfulness is also not transcendental meditation. It is attention to the present moment.

When mindfulness is tied to spiritual practices of meditation, it should be compatible with your worldview. In the Christian faith, trustful surrender to God leads to mindfulness. The invisible God is ever present. Focusing on the present moment often brings awareness of God's presence. This is how we "let go and let God"—trusting him in every moment.

In the Christian faith, filling the mind with the mind of Christ is the focus and can be added to the breath focus. The more you fill your mind with the mind of Christ, the more peace you will find. Furthermore, when you pay attention to God's presence, you worry less about your future and can set your mind on the promises and goodness of God. This shuts out distraction, diminishes worry, and allows you to listen in the moment to God.

So when contemplative practices are used, elements of spirituality of any kind must be acknowledged. Make the practice of mindfulness true to your spiritual beliefs or simply practice being more present in the moment. Both can help you manage stress and reduce pain.

Other Ways to Reduce Stress

Here are several other ways to reduce stress that you may have overlooked.

Sing

A church leader once asked me (Linda) to come and talk about stress management. One of the first things I asked those in the audience was, "How many of you sing in the choir?" Several hands went up. Then I said, "Did you know that choir singing is a stress reducer? Robustly singing is good not only for the soul and the spirit but also for the body."[20] In fact, when I embarrass my children by belting out a tune in the car, I tell them that Mom is reducing stress. Yes, they are embarrassed, but I feel better!

Singing releases endorphins in the brain and the hormone oxytocin, which helps with anxiety and bonding. Singing relaxes the mind and the body. It slows the pulse and heart rate, lowers blood pressure, and decreases stress hormones. It is a natural tranquilizer that soothes the nerves and makes us feel better. It distracts us and touches our emotions. So embrace singing in the shower, in your car, at home, or wherever. It doesn't matter if you can carry a tune. Just sing. Belt out a song, join a choir, do karaoke, create an ensemble, and sing to de-stress.

Take a Time-Out

Many of us deal with stress due to relationship difficulties. Just like stressed children can calm down with a time-out, adults can do the same. If you find yourself getting worked up over an argument, conflict, or conversation, take a five-minute time-out, do some deep breathing, and refocus your thoughts on working through the issue. When you feel relaxed and you can think again, reengage.

Or use a time-out from distractions. Unplug from devices. Get off social media. Spend a few moments alone to recenter your thoughts and refocus on what is important in life.

Connect with People

Sometimes we need a time-out from people; other times we need to force ourselves to make social connections. Maybe you haven't thought of getting out of the house and being with people as stress relief, but it can work for some people. Go for coffee, see a movie, go to church or temple, and so forth. Anything that gets you interacting with others and diverts attention away from pain can be relaxing. Sometimes sitting alone in your house or apartment can create more stress.

Assess Your Goals and Make Them Realistic

Sometimes we are stressed because we have unrealistic goals. When it comes to chronic pain, you can reduce your pain and increase your function and quality of life if your goals are realistic. Discuss your expectations with the team that works with you regarding pain. It helps to be on the same page and working toward the same goals. Stress can be brought on when you and those helping you with pain have different expectations as to pain management.

Laugh

Researchers actually did a study on how well humor relieves chronic pain because of the stress relief it provides.[21] They went to a nursing home and implemented a humor therapy program. The outcome was an effective nonpharmacological intervention for chronic pain. Laughter *is* good medicine. Humor can be healing.

You may be familiar with the story of journalist and peace advocate Norman Cousins.[22] He was diagnosed with a degenerative and debilitating disease, ankylosing spondylitis. The prognosis for this disease is grim, and he was given very bad news as to becoming disabled and eventually dying. Cousins decided to check himself into a hotel and rent hours' worth of Marx Brothers comedy and *Candid Camera* episodes. He laughed and laughed, which enabled him to sleep and his body to heal. He lived another twenty-six years and became the poster child for studying the effects of laughter on the physiology of the body.

Laughter produces endorphins, boosts immunity, lowers stress hormones, and decreases pain. When you laugh, your pain threshold increases.[23] While chronic pain is no laughing matter, laughter can be one of the tools used to keep chronic pain manageable.

Participate in Leisure Activities

Sedentary behaviors such as watching television for hours do not help a person with chronic pain.[24] With chronic pain, it is necessary to build strength and flexibility. Both can be done through leisure activities. An entire field called recreation therapy helps people incorporate play and fun into daily living. Sports can be adapted to disabilities and limitations a person may experience. A sport such as golf may be possible if you work with someone on your swing to eliminate sources of pain. (We will discuss this in more detail in chapter 18.)

The point is that leisure activities that get you up and moving and interacting with other people can be a tremendous pain reliever. Why? Because movement and activity relieve stress and take your mind off pain. Work with an occupational therapist or a recreational therapist for ways to add leisure activities into your life.

Spiritual Resources and Rest

Resources to cope with stress can be depleted over time. People let us down, control is elusive, and time moves forward. But a person's faith is an unlimited resource that can be continuously accessed.

In times of stress, faith can be incredibly important. Help comes from God, who is ever present. God is not only our present help in times of trouble but also the God of more than enough, El Shaddai. Call on him. Ask him to supply your need. In our culture of self-sufficiency, we often forget to access the endless supply of provision we have through our faith. Instead, we rely on ourselves and eventually feel stressed and exhausted.

If you are tired and stressed, schedule time with God for refreshment and relaxation. He is the one who nourishes us as the Living Water and the Bread of Life. Intimate time with God is our greatest resource to managing stress. The promise is that if we dwell in the shelter of the Most High, we will rest in his shadow (Ps. 91:1). Right now, a little rest may be needed to move you from stressed to refreshed.

17

Change Your Lifestyle, Change Your Pain

Don't look for the big, quick improvement. Seek the small improvement one day at a time. That's the only way it happens—and when it happens, it lasts.

John Wooden

Lifestyle is a factor in the management of many diseases and conditions. The way a person lives and the habits they develop can make pain worse or better. Attending to your lifestyle may improve your overall sense of well-being and be part of those marginal gains necessary to live beyond pain.

Alcohol

The use of alcohol to dull pain can be traced back to ancient times, when wine was mixed with myrrh or gall. It was used to mitigate pain for those who were sentenced to die by crucifixion and is referenced in the biblical account of Jesus's crucifixion.

While alcohol is no longer used in this fashion, people often use it to self-medicate both physical and emotional pain. It is readily available and used as a coping mechanism for stress, albeit not a good one. The National Institute on Alcohol Abuse and Alcoholism estimates that 28 percent of chronic pain sufferers use alcohol to mask pain.[1] The Dietary Guidelines for Americans state that moderate drinking is no more than one drink a day for women and two drinks a day for men.[2] Otherwise, you are not considered a moderate drinker.

In general, drinking to medicate pain is not a good option. First, alcohol and medications don't mix well together. Many prescription medications have an alcohol warning on them. Drinking and taking aspirin and acetaminophen, two common over-the-counter medications for pain relief, can affect the liver or promote gastric bleeding. Cardiac problems, respiratory problems, and potential alcohol poisoning are possible when benzodiazepines, often used to treat anxiety, are mixed with alcohol. And, of course, mixing alcohol and opioids can be a deadly combination.

Here is a story of a woman who never thought about mixing alcohol with a prescription drug. She was in chronic pain because of an undiagnosed condition. At first, she wasn't sure why she was having excruciating pain. Eventually, she was diagnosed with kidney stones and prescribed tramadol. The physician never asked her history and thus didn't know she drank alcohol every day. He told her to take the medication as needed and prescribed thirty pills. But tramadol can have life-threatening consequences when it is mixed with alcohol. She was not informed that this drug has a black box warning, the most serious warning from the FDA that states the drug's side effects may be dangerous and even lead to overdose and death. Her daily drinking was an important fact that was overlooked. Fortunately, when she realized the danger, she stopped drinking alcohol.

Second, when pain is involved, it is easy to exceed moderate drinking and use alcohol to escape pain and life. The more a person drinks, the more they build up a tolerance to the analgesic effect, so they have to drink more to cover the pain. Then if they decide they are drinking too much and try to stop, withdrawal from chronic alcohol use can increase pain sensitivity.

Alcohol affects the central nervous system so that pain perception is lessened, but the alcohol itself does not have any pain-relieving properties. And using alcohol to cover pain can lead to addiction. So if you are using alcohol to relieve your pain, talk to your physician about better ways to control your pain.

Smoking

One of my (Linda's) favorite Muppet movies contains a line delivered by Pepe the king prawn. My children remember this line because of his French accent. During one scene, he turns to his Muppet friends and says, "Smoking it not good for you, okay?" He's right—especially when it comes to pain. Smoking is often used to manage and distract a person from pain, but it is noteworthy that smoking is more prevalent in the pain population than in the general population.[3] In fact, the data indicates that heavy smokers report more pain locations and an increase in pain intensity compared to people who never smoked.[4] While we can't say with certainty that quitting smoking will improve your pain because pain clinic patients have low success rates when it comes to smoking cessation, we do know that smoking is a major risk factor for cardiovascular disease[5] and has been shown to be associated with mortality among people with chronic pain.[6] This link to mortality should be a motivator to quit. Smoking cessation is not easy for most people, though, because nicotine is highly addictive. In order to quit, you will likely need an intense smoking cessation program.

Weight

Being overweight makes it difficult to function in many areas of everyday life. Overweight people report 20 percent greater pain than people of normal weight. The percentages of pain complaints rise when the weight of a person increases.[7] Weight often limits movement, and a person becomes deconditioned and may reduce their physical activity. They don't play ball with their grandchildren or take walks in the park. This lack of movement makes pain worse. More pain is also felt due to the increased weight-bearing on joints.[8] Every extra pound of weight a person carries exerts an extra four pounds of pressure on the knees.[9] So, for example, ten pounds of additional weight exerts an additional forty pounds of pressure on the knee joints.

In some cases, chronic pain prompts weight gain. Many factors involved in chronic pain—sleep problems, medication side effects, sedentary lifestyle, and so on—contribute to weight gain.

Since weight can both aggravate pain and lead to pain, weight loss can help in the fight to manage pain. Good weight loss programs include dietary help and exercise. (Exercise is considered in chapter 18.) Slow and steady win the race when it comes to losing pounds.

In his eulogy for Hall of Famer Moses Malone, Charles Barkley, who was affectionately known as the "Round Mound of Rebound," told a great story of how to use small goals to work toward something greater.[10] He shared that when he was drafted by the Philadelphia 76ers, he weighed three hundred pounds. He was frustrated because he wasn't getting the desired playing time and the opportunity to contribute as he felt he could. So he confided in his veteran team member, Moses Malone. "Mo, I'm really struggling. What can I do? Give me some advice." Malone encouraged Barkley to lose ten pounds. The rookie committed to losing weight, and through changing his diet and working with Malone before and after practice, he lost not just ten but fifteen pounds in one week.

He went to Malone for affirmation. "Lose ten more," Malone said. Barkley again disciplined himself and began to have increased energy and stamina as well as increased playing time. When he lost ten more pounds, he again went to Malone. "Lose ten more. Give me ten more." This happened again and again until Barkley had lost fifty pounds.

Barkley went on to have a Hall of Fame career, averaging over twenty-two points and nearly twelve rebounds per game. He credits the man he would later call Dad, Moses Malone, with helping him focus, get healthy, and thrive in his career.

Later, Barkley asked, "Mo, why didn't you just tell me to lose fifty pounds?" The answer was a wise one: "Because if I told you to lose it all at once, you would have never done it."

Losing weight, eating healthy, and exercising are hard to do. If these were easy changes, we would all have quick success. The key is to set realistic goals and stay motivated toward creating a healthier lifestyle.

On the journey of trying to create a healthier you, celebrate small victories—remember the concept of marginal gains. But make sure that when you celebrate, the rewards you use are not foods that promote weight gain or inflammation. Instead, choose rewards that encourage healthy living, such as a massage, bath salts, a new book, hand weights, money toward a vacation, tickets to a game, and so on. You need to break the association between food and reward for long-term maintenance of weight loss.

To help improve your pain, get as close as possible to your ideal weight. Joining a program such as Weight Watchers can be very helpful because it involves accountability and interaction with others. Having support is critical to sustained weight loss. So find a weight-loss program that helps you change your lifestyle into one that can be sustained over time, or find your own Mo to encourage you along the journey.

Hydration

Our bodies need an internal balance of water and electrolytes to function properly. Given that our bodies are about 60 percent water, to stay well, we need to pay attention to our fluid intake. Hydration helps the heart, kidneys, digestion, and cognition.

We lose fluid a variety of ways throughout the day—through exercise and sweating; through frequent urination due to diseases such as diabetes and medications that increase urination (e.g., blood pressure diuretics such as hydrochlorothiazide); through vomiting and/or diarrhea due to illness; and so forth. Signs of dehydration often include thirst, fatigue, dry skin, muscle cramps, infrequent urination, dizziness, and cognitive changes. An easy way to check your hydration is to look at the color of your urine. If it is dark yellow, cloudy, or smells bad (not due to something you ate such as asparagus), drink more fluids.

Water helps blood circulate. When you don't get enough water, the oxygen-rich blood flowing to your brain can bring on pain. When the body loses fluid faster than it is replenished, a dehydration headache can occur. The brain temporarily contracts from fluid loss. This triggers pain receptors in the membranes surrounding the brain called the meninges, resulting in a headache. Hydration helps the brain return to its normal state.[11] Hydration can ease pain and in some cases relieve it.

How much water do you need each day? Experts recommend you drink at least half your body weight in ounces of water each day. So, for example, if you weigh 150 pounds, you should drink 75 ounces of water a day. You can also get water by eating fruits and vegetables. If you drink coffee and alcohol, remember that these are diuretics and promote urination and fluid loss.

Diet

Food is an important substance for every chemical process in the body. If you want to function better, you need to eat better. The saying "You are what you eat" especially applies to pain. Food choices matter. Food affects the brain and the microbiome, influencing both inflammation and mood.

When your body stays in an inflammatory state, it can damage healthy cells and organs, leading to pain in muscles, tissues, and joints. Because pain is often tied to inflammation, an anti-inflammatory diet is helpful in reducing pain. Certain foods can promote or shut down the biochemical process of inflammation.

William Welches, pain management specialist at the Cleveland Clinic, notes that patients who eat a strict vegan or Mediterranean diet can reduce inflammation and ease pain symptoms. Along with exercise and stress management, this type of eating helps control insulin and cholesterol and reduce inflammation.[12] Here are his three general recommendations:

1. Choose eight or nine servings of vegetables each day (a few of those could be fruit servings instead). The best vegetables are the cruciferous ones (broccoli, brussels sprouts, cabbage, cauliflower, etc.).
2. Limit dairy and refined grains. Avoid simple carbohydrates and refined sugar. Simple carbohydrates can promote inflammation. Instead, eat whole grains such as barley, buckwheat, oats, quinoa, brown rice, rye, spelt, and wheat.
3. Avoid red meat. Substitute fish for red meat. Chicken is not harmful but is also not beneficial in the inflammatory fight.

Generally speaking, the staples of the Mediterranean diet are whole fruits (especially berries), dark-green leafy vegetables, nuts, legumes, and whole grains. The foods you want to avoid are processed junk foods with low nutritional value, sodas, simple sugars such as high-fructose corn syrup, processed meat, white bread and pasta, and foods high in refined carbohydrates. Oils such as extra-virgin olive oil and canola oil are healthier than butter.

The Cleveland Clinic also suggests spices and supplements to help nourish the body and fight inflammation: turmeric, ginger, fish oil, glucosamine, chondroitin, proteolytic enzymes, boswellia, and white willow bark. We would add devil's claw. Always discuss supplements with your physician due to possible interactions with other medical conditions you may have or medications you might be taking.[13]

Others who treat pain advocate for a high-protein diet that avoids carbohydrates and high-glycemic foods.[14] People on opioids can gain weight due to a poor nutritional diet and a preference for sweet foods that is related to how opioids regulate sugar intake and how sugar intake affects the endogenous opiate system. Because of a diet high in sugar, blood sugar can be unstable and cause hypoglycemia.[15] Eating a high-protein, low-carbohydrate diet may help with weight loss and hypoglycemia. Protein derivatives are endogenous pain relievers, build muscle, activate glucagon (which blocks glucose storage as fat), and decrease inflammation.

If you need extra help to make dietary changes, work with a registered dietitian who can review your food choices and create an eating plan that will help your pain. Journal what you eat and replace high-calorie foods with low-calorie choices, such as carrots and hummus in place of chips. Build a support system to keep you motivated and moving forward. Diet may not fix your chronic pain, but it will help you manage and possibly prevent inflammation, reducing pain.

Sleep

Sleep problems are a reliable predictor of pain.[16] Over half of people who attend pain clinics report they have trouble sleeping.[17] Sleep and pain are reciprocally related. Chronic pain can cause sleep problems, and sleep problems can cause pain.

Scientists can't fully explain why we need sleep, but humans and all animals do. Sleep is restorative to the body. It helps the immune system and cognitive functions. A lack of sleep disrupts many of the physiological processes in the body. Stress rises, appetite increases, metabolism slows down, and cognitive function is impaired. Sleep deprivation can disrupt endogenous opioid systems in the body and make you more prone to persistent pain.[18]

The sleep cycle is repeated a number of times during the night. You start with lighter stages of sleep, then go into deeper sleep and into rapid eye movement (REM) sleep, where dreaming occurs. When chronic pain is present, it can disrupt the sleep cycle, preventing you from falling back asleep or waking you up too soon.

One reason falling asleep is so problematic is because your brain is more aware of pain when all the other distractions of the day stop. However, this is when you can practice relaxation techniques to manage your pain. Here are a few more ideas:

- If you begin to worry, write down your concerns so that you can think about them tomorrow. If you are a person of faith, reminding yourself to trust God for tomorrow can calm your spirit and mind.
- Try focusing on a nonpainful part of your body and imagine that part of the body warming. This mind exercise moves your focus away from the source of your pain.
- Mentally, separate the painful part of your body from the rest of your body. For instance, imagine your back sitting in a chair across the room and staying there.
- If a part of your body feels hot from pain, focus on the sensation of heat instead of the pain.
- In your mind, imagine injecting a numbing agent into the part of your body that hurts. Or imagine a soothing ice pack on the area.
- Turn off screens and electronics, as the lights wake up the brain and mimic daylight.
- Don't exercise too close to bedtime, as this disrupts sleep.
- Purchase a good mattress and pillow and make your bed comfortable. A pillow should support the natural curve

of your neck. If you are a side sleeper, use a thicker pillow than someone who sleeps on their back, as your head should be positioned in the middle of your shoulders.

- Avoid stomach sleeping. This is especially bad for neck pain.
- Avoid caffeine late in the day, as it remains in the body for hours.
- Avoid fatty or sugary foods before bed. Milk can be sleep promoting.
- Avoid alcohol, as it might help you fall asleep but tends to cause sleep disruptions the rest of the night.
- Avoid napping during the day.
- Avoid staying in bed during the day.
- Avoid stressful activities prior to bedtime.
- Stop smoking. It is a risk factor for sleep apnea and causes difficulty falling asleep and leads to waking earlier than desired.
- Add a soothing sound, like the sound of waves, or use a fan.
- Cool down the room, as we all sleep better when the temperature is cooler. Try different temperatures to see what works best for you.
- Use the bedroom only for sleep and sex, or you will associate sleep with other activities.
- Darken the room. Consider light-blocking curtains.
- Untreated depression can result in early morning waking, so seek treatment if needed.
- If you are still struggling with falling asleep after twenty minutes or so, get out of bed and do a nonstimulating activity until you become sleepy.
- If you are not refreshed or feel exhausted after you've had a full night of rest, consult your physician about sleep-disturbed breathing or sleep apnea.

- Try to go to bed and wake up at the same times. This will help regulate your body systems toward sleep.
- Develop a nighttime routine such as reading, prayer time, or journaling. This will help calm your mind down and inform your body that it is time to sleep.
- If you struggle with insomnia, consider hiding the clock. Watching time pass creates anxiety and another hurdle for falling back asleep.

When sleep problems are based in chronic medical problems, they need to be addressed with a physician. Problems such as restless leg syndrome and sleep apnea, in which breathing stops for about ten seconds or airflow is reduced, wake the brain. Also know that opioid pain medications have been associated with sleep apnea.[19]

We advise that nonmedication sleep approaches be tried first. If the preceding suggestions and the relaxation techniques discussed in chapter 16 do not work, consult with your physician about sleep medications.

To better control pain, make lifestyle changes. While these changes are not always easy, the benefits for better health are significant. List each lifestyle change discussed in this chapter. Do a self-evaluation of each area. Then take a step to change one thing. For example, you could drink more water in your day. As you are successful with one thing, you can tackle another. The goal is to make changes in each of the lifestyle areas as a way to decrease pain and improve function.

18

The Importance of Exercise and Movement

You just do it. You force yourself to get up. You force yourself
to put one foot before the other, you refuse to let it get to you.
You fight. You cry. You curse. Then you go about the business of living. That's how I've done it. There's no other way.

Elizabeth Taylor

When talking about ways to manage or eliminate pain, exercise
and movement top the list of many pain managers. Yes, exercise
is a lifestyle change, but because it is so important, it deserves
its own chapter. Moving in ways that are enjoyable and inspiring
can build confidence and lead to a more pleasant life. Pain limits
movement, and so people in pain often have to gently push against
those limits in ways that are reasonable but sometimes challenging.
People in pain have good days and bad, which affects their ability
to move and exercise.

Intuitively, people think they should rest and be inactive to relieve their pain. But more and more we are finding that exercise

has many benefits, not only for chronic pain but also for overall physical and mental health and functioning.[1] When considering exercise and movement, always assess safety and talk to your physician. Goals need to be reasonable and monitored. Let's face it, even when we know that exercise can help, it is often hard to do and keep doing. It requires motivation. But it may be one of the best ways to improve your life and pain.

The Cochrane reviews are systematic reviews of primary research in health care and policies. Basically, this group is responsible for reviewing research conducted in an area such as exercise and pain and providing conclusions based on all the studies that have been done. Regarding movement and pain, several studies noted positive results with exercise regarding functioning and quality of life. A few studies showed improvement in pain severity. Exercise does not worsen pain. The most reported side effect was muscle pain or soreness that subsided over time.[2]

While more research is needed on the impact of exercise on chronic pain, studies seem to suggest that exercise and physical activity have few adverse effects and improve pain and quality of life. The general thinking is to keep active. The more you can take charge of your health through movement, the better.

Exercise increases sleep quality, energy levels, blood flow, and tissue oxygenation, and it can improve cognition. It can also increase serotonin and other endorphins, helping with depression and neuromodulation. It can increase the production of endogenous opioids and help mood.[3] Exercise can also increase strength, improve posture, and optimize the skeletal framework in which the other systems in the body operate. It can increase balance and flexibility, reducing the risk of falls, injury, and additional pain. Certain types of resistance exercise can support bone and cartilage related to joints.[4] Exercise can help you live better with pain and in some cases help you leave pain behind altogether.

Physical activity can take many forms—structured classes, gym-based programs, home exercises, and activities of daily living. It can vary in intensity, duration, and type (think aerobic and anaerobic). It can take place in a group, be individually performed, and be driven by various levels of motivation. Most important, it can be adapted to you and is something that you can do to take charge of your life. Always check with a physician to determine what might be beneficial in your situation.

Generally speaking, the best way to approach exercise is to do it gradually. The idea is to break the cycle of inactivity and deconditioning. You do this by gradually increasing the length of time and the intensity of the activity.

It has been said in medicine that the best exercise you can prescribe for a patient is the one the patient will do. I (James) am cautious about this phrase because I don't want it to seem glib or be misunderstood as condescension. What it means is that increasing movement is vital, but you have to start where you are. Getting out of bed and sitting for fifteen minutes, if that is where you are, is as much of a victory as walking to the mailbox or jogging three miles might be for someone else.

In addition, the best exercises you can do are not necessarily protocol driven. Many times a dozen specific exercises are given to a patient based on their general diagnosis, such as a rotator cuff tear or osteoarthritis of the knee. While these exercises do provide benefit and should be done to target areas that need restoration, the results can sometimes be limited. The problem is that dysfunction of a shoulder or a knee doesn't occur in isolation from the rest of the body. Improving mobility, flexibility, and strength in the entire body improves connection, blood flow, and neural relationships with the dysfunctional part and helps it heal. So whether you are performing exercises provided by your physician or physical therapist or starting on your own in a pool or with chair exercises, it is important to involve your whole body as much as you can.

The following are exercises that you may find especially helpful when dealing with pain.

Yoga

There are many references to yoga in the pain literature. This is a practice that originates from Hindu spirituality. It includes breath control, meditation, and the use of specific body postures. Yoga incorporates stretching, flexibility, and isometric strength training (holding certain poses with no movement against a resistance).

Yoga is not an established religion but is considered a spiritual path. According to Rajiv Malhotra, author of *Being Different: An Indian Challenge to Western Universalism*, "yoga's metaphysics center on the quest to attain liberation from one's conditioning caused by past karma. Karma includes the baggage from prior lives, underscoring the importance of reincarnation." Malhotra, in his opinion as a Hindu, goes on to say that yoga cannot be done from a Christian perspective.[5]

Because of yoga's spiritual underpinnings, there is debate in the Christian community about its practice. Some maintain that a person can practice yoga apart from its spiritual roots; others say that spiritual ideas are embedded in the postures and the practice. It is not the purpose of this book to debate this practice. If you feel comfortable with it, know that yoga can help with pain management by increasing strength and flexibility. If you have concerns about the practice in light of your worldview, there are alternatives, including Pilates.

Pilates

Pilates is a low-impact type of exercise that focuses on core strength and flexibility using multiple muscle groups. Similar to yoga, it also focuses on posture, balance, breathing, and body movements.

Pilates was originally developed by Joseph Pilates as an exercise program for injured dancers and soldiers. This system of exercise can be done by both beginners and those who regularly exercise. Pilates can incorporate a special apparatus designed to improve physical strength, flexibility, and posture, or it can be done with only a mat on the floor in the comfort of your home and guided by an app. Pilates classes are also offered in many health clubs.

Muscles and joints often accommodate for weakness in areas of pain. Pilates works on the muscular support system of the body to offload joints and reduce pain. It has been shown to be effective in people with chronic low-back pain[6] and other pain conditions.

Pilates brought me (Linda) back to health after my microdiscectomy. While my back surgery was considered a success, I was given no postsurgical instructions as to how to reengage in life without fear of injuring myself. I was also in pain.

With the consent of my doctor (you need to be cleared to exercise) and after a period of healing, I began a Pilates program at the local YMCA. It made a difference in terms of bringing me back to health and helping me have a full and active life again. I started slowly, under guidance, and eventually exchanged achiness and stiffness for increased balance, flexibility, and core strength. It improved my overall well-being and was a stress reducer. It took my focus off the pain and put it on building my core strength.

Again, always check with your physician because those with herniated discs, unstable blood pressure, risk of blood clots, and osteoarthritis may need other forms of movement. Adjustments might need to be made for those with diabetes and especially diabetic retinopathy, as you may need to avoid certain movements. Women who are pregnant may also need to adjust some movements. For arthritis, Pilates can help with symptoms and keep joints flexible.[7]

Tai Chi

The martial art of tai chi is rooted in Chinese medicine. It has become a mind-body adjunctive practice used in treating or preventing health problems. It is about achieving physical and emotional balance and has been shown to be effective in reducing pain. For example, a recent study at Tufts University found tai chi to be more effective for symptom improvement in patients with fibromyalgia than aerobic exercise.[8] The study also noted improvements in anxiety, depression, and self-efficacy.

Tai chi involves slow and deliberate movements. It is often referred to as meditation in motion. It is a form of movement that places less emphasis on the joints and muscles as compared to more strenuous forms of exercise due to the way it is performed and includes deep breathing. There are several forms, with some focusing on health and others on self-defense.

The benefits of this exercise are improved lower and upper body strength, flexibility, balance, and some aerobic conditioning. As with any form of exercise, check with your physician if you have limiting musculoskeletal problems or are taking medications that can make you dizzy or lightheaded.

The spiritual roots of tai chi as a religious practice come from Taoism. Taoism and western religions are based on very different worldviews. So again, if the spiritual origins of this practice matter to you, choose accordingly, but add exercise and movement to your life.

A good way to begin exercising is to use low-impact equipment such as balance balls and resistance bands. You can download fitness apps to be used in the privacy of your own home. Water aerobics classes take the stress off joints and muscles. As a side note, when I (Linda) was working with obese patients who wanted to exercise but not deal with wearing a bathing suit in public, I arranged for a local YMCA to open early so my patients could have a private water aerobics class. They were motivated to attend, and they bonded with one another. They worked hard and reported improvement in pain and other areas of their lives.

When it comes to exercise, having a partner or others involved helps keep you accountable. It is too easy to make excuses when no one is challenging you to keep moving.

You can find many ways to increase movement without a formal exercise class or going to a gym, if those activities do not work in your schedule. Participate in a community event such as walking for breast cancer, or add movement by playing Wii, Xbox, or PlayStation dance games with your children. They can be fun and geared to your own abilities. Whatever you choose, check with your physician first, stay positive, pace yourself, and keep moving forward. Don't be sedentary or take on too much. Find something you enjoy and include others to make exercise a part of your lifestyle. Exercise and movement are ways to take control of your pain.

19

When You Need More Help

You may not control all the events that happen to you, but
you can decide not to be reduced by them.

Maya Angelou

There are times in our lives when we feel stuck and may need help
from someone who is more objective—and trained to move us from
stuck to unstuck. A pain specialist or therapist who understands
chronic pain can be a boost to moving you forward.

Accepting a referral to talk therapy is not easy for people in
pain. The implication is that pain is all in your head and that you
are somehow crazy. But by now, we hope you don't believe that. You
can see how complicated it is to deal with pain and how making
changes in many areas of your life can help you live beyond pain.
At times, people need help making these changes and focusing on
quality of life and overall well-being.

Having someone listen to you, empathize, and legitimize your
pain can be extremely helpful. Developing a trusting relationship with someone who will give you acceptance, comfort, and

reassurance can improve your life and keep you moving forward. Social support is known to help heal and improve pain.[1]

Psychotherapy can help teach relaxation methods; bring accountability to exercise and lifestyle changes; help you discover ways to live with pain while effectively reducing harm; and help you deal with thoughts, moods, and relationships. In some cases, therapy can help a person find meaning in pain and prevent depression and even suicide. The belief that improvement is possible is essential to living well.

Certain types of therapies are especially effective for chronic pain and can help with pain interference and mood.[2] One is acceptance and commitment therapy (ACT), and another is cognitive behavioral therapy (CBT). Both ACT and CBT emphasize the present moment and are considered evidence-based therapies for chronic pain.

Acceptance and Commitment Therapy (ACT)

ACT is a type of therapy that is based on the idea that it is the struggle with pain that causes suffering. The approach encourages you to reduce the influence of thoughts and emotions on actions. ACT emphasizes disconnecting from the struggle of pain and finding meaning through your values and goals in order to build psychological flexibility. Psychological flexibility is your ability to be aware of and accept thoughts and feelings. Instead of struggling against thoughts and feelings, choose a direction consistent with your values and goals.[3] Pain may be present, but you choose how much it interferes with your life. Then you can commit to action that will take you to your goals, based on your values. This is a behavioral therapy focused on behavior change that is accomplished through committed action.[4] It uses methods such as exposure, behavioral activation, skills training, and mindfulness and has been shown to increase physical and social functioning and decrease pain-related medical visits.[5]

The acceptance piece is important, because pain acceptance is a better predictor of pain outcomes than pain severity.[6] Acceptance does not mean you give in to pain and are helpless. Instead, when you accept the reality of pain and stop fighting against it, you can choose what to do with it.

Following acceptance, you commit to behavior change. You change behavior by changing the way you experience thoughts, feelings, and sensations. You notice your pain thoughts without necessarily acting on them, believing them, or being controlled by them. By exposing yourself to the emotions and sensations of pain, you gradually reduce fear and behave in ways more in accordance with your goals. Pain and its sensations will come and go. In the process, you learn to detach from old mind scripts that are negative concerning pain. What you value (e.g., a better life) and how you act need to be consistent.

Cognitive Behavioral Therapy (CBT)

Brain-imaging studies actually show the impact of using cognitive behavioral therapy (CBT) with pain experiences. The volume in the regions of the brain associated with pain control actually increases after sessions of CBT. Mind-set interventions for pain relief make a difference. No matter where you feel pain in your body, it is processed in the central nervous system, the brain, and the spinal cord. Remember, these things are highly responsive to the way we think.

The aim of CBT is to reduce pain behaviors (e.g., avoidance of activities, moaning, asking for help, etc.) and increase healthy behavior (e.g., increased movement and exercise, etc.). Because this type of therapy addresses your thoughts and teaches you to change your thinking by making thoughts more rational and true to the moment, it helps you challenge inaccurate and negative thoughts. It uses approaches such as cognitive restructuring, shaping, gradual exercise, and so forth. These approaches focus on changing negative beliefs, thoughts, emotions, and behaviors that keep a person stuck. They also target behaviors that will help a person gradually engage in more functional behavior. For chronic pain, goals are typically to improve movement, social skills, pain coping, and other areas of functioning. The focus is to take charge of pain and manage it by being more active and problem-solving. In CBT, functioning related to pain can be addressed even if the pain remains unchanged. Thus, CBT can have an effect on reducing pain and aid functioning.[7]

Mindfulness-Based Stress Reduction

Another widely used therapy for pain management is a third mind-body therapy called mindfulness-based stress reduction (MBSR).[8] It was mentioned in chapter 16 as it relates to mindfulness as a technique for focused attention.

The founder of this therapy, Jon Kabat-Zinn, based the mindfulness component of the therapy on Buddhist practice adapted to mental health. Mindfulness in MBSR is taught as a secular practice and teaches people to relate to their pain. It is based on the idea that we have a choice as to how we respond to experiences. We can become aware of our habits and reactions and choose a different path.

This approach trains the brain to lessen experiences of discomfort and possibly eliminate them. It typically uses guided meditation, yoga, and breathing exercises. A goal is to choose to deal with pain and relieve suffering by turning down the volume on pain amplifiers. The idea is based on the notion that pain reduction occurs by adopting an attitude of detached observation toward the pain sensations when you become aware of them. Separating the physical sensations from the emotional and thinking experiences of pain helps reduce pain. Distraction from pain, coping strategies toward pain, and heightened awareness of pain sensation lead to behavior change.

Included in this approach is a "body scan" in which you bring awareness to all parts of your body. Breathing is used to calm your mind. Healthy distraction is used. The focus is to pay attention to pain and be curious about it while accepting its existence. Home practice has been tied to better outcomes.[9] This can be practiced using a secular approach to mindfulness that is based on focused attention or a Christian approach to mindfulness in which awareness of God's eternal presence is emphasized.

Any therapeutic approach is delivered through the worldview of the practitioner. Therefore, it is important to ask about a therapist's worldview and be comfortable with the person delivering the therapy. We have highlighted the three most discussed therapies in the chronic pain literature. Many more therapies can be used to help people in pain. Whatever therapy you use, you should always work with a mental health professional who is trained and licensed.

20

Complementary and Alternative Approaches to Pain Management

Any doctor can hang a shingle that says "I treat pain." Look for doctors who are board-certified in pain medicine or who did a fellowship in something pain-related.

Michelle Crouch

A number of approaches to pain management are considered complementary or alternative. If they are nonmainstreamed but used with conventional medicine, they are considered complementary. If they are used in place of conventional medicine, they are considered alternative.

Integrative medicine is an attempt to bring complementary and conventional approaches together in a way that improves health and wellness. Practices we have already discussed—including deep breathing, progressive muscle relaxation, biofeedback, mindfulness, yoga, tai chi, and massage—are examples of more well-known complementary approaches to pain management. This chapter discusses a few more approaches used to treat pain. We have chosen not to cover dietary supplements because of the potential interactions they can have with some prescription medications. Always discuss dietary supplements with your health-care provider before you decide to add them to your treatment plan.

In fact, if you decide to use any complementary or alternative approach, check with your health-care provider first to make sure it is safe for you and your unique pain presentation. Always remember that "natural" doesn't necessarily mean safe. Learn as much as you can about an approach. Many complementary and alternative treatments remain under study. Be mindful of the fact that people with a financial incentive often sponsor research to support the use of their products. So have a scientific eye when looking at how effective certain treatments will be. If you aren't sure, print out a copy of a study and take it to your health-care provider. And don't be afraid to ask for a second opinion. Finally, make sure the person providing the treatment is experienced and well trained.

Acupuncture

Acupuncture is an ancient healing art that uses fine needles precisely inserted in the skin to affect a person's health and pain. As is the case with other healing arts, we don't completely understand the mechanisms at play with acupuncture, which has been used, literally, for millennia. However, various Western studies suggest that acupuncture works based on the gate control theory of pain discussed earlier. This theory essentially says that there are places on the pain pathways that open or close the gates to pain. What is thought to occur with acupuncture is that, by placing needles in precise locations, neuromodulators are stimulated that close the gate on the pain message.[1] In other words, the brain doesn't receive or fully translate the message trying to be sent as pain. It is hypothesized that this may be because of changes at the molecular level that result in pain relief.[2] As a result, acupuncture is thought to stimulate the body's own healing.

Proponents say that acupuncture has to be done safely and with caution, especially if you have a pacemaker, skin problems, and other conditions that could be affected. Skin infections can occur if needles are not clean. Usually multiple treatments are needed for more enduring effects. It is wise to check with your physician to make sure this type of procedure is compatible with your medical history and current medical conditions. That said, be aware that there is controversy in terms of the effectiveness of acupuncture to relieve pain.[3]

Many studies have looked at the idea of a placebo affecting pain. Does the belief that something *may* work *make* it work? Is acupuncture simply an elaborate placebo? Some say yes. The argument usually hinges on the question as to the realness of the acupuncture points. Skeptics cite a large body of studies that do not demonstrate clinical benefit to acupuncture and take the position that rigorous science does not support the claims made as to the effectiveness of acupuncture.[4]

However, those who believe acupuncture stimulates a physiological response say it is more than a placebo. They use several studies to support their side of the argument[5] that show a physiologic response in the central serotonergic system,[6] in the endogenous opioid system,[7] and with viserosomatic reflexes.[8] Cochrane review studies found acupuncture to be effective in treating common pain disorders. There was moderate support for acupuncture reducing the frequency of migraines after six treatments and being as effective as drugs taken that prevent migranes.[9] Similar support has also been found for the use of acupuncture for tension headaches.[10] There is low- to moderate-level evidence that acupuncture improves pain and stiffness in those with fibromyalgia compared to those who received no treatment, yet there is also moderate-level evidence that acupuncture does not differ from sham acupuncture in reducing pain or other symptoms associated with fibromyalgia.[11] Wherever you stand on this issue, it is clear that acupuncture will continue to be a popular area of study because it is considered a noninvasive treatment with few side effects.

In clinical practice, acupuncture is well tolerated by most patients. The needles are exquisitely thin and felt in the skin only momentarily, if at all. Once a needle is in place, people sometimes report a tingling sensation or a mild achiness, but the discomfort is usually mild and, for some, well worth it.

An important consideration when deciding if acupuncture is right for you is to have a clear understanding of what is causing your pain. I (Linda) mentioned before that I used acupuncture as an attempt to ease my chronic pain before I knew its cause. Fortunately for me, the physician performing the acupuncture realized the source of my pain and knew acupuncture could not cure it. I did have temporary relief with acupuncture. This is only my experience, which is why you should be aware of the scientific findings and consult a physician about your unique condition. We do know that if you believe something works or can help you, it can change your pain perception. If this is an approach you decide to use, find a certified provider.[12]

Regenerative Medicine

In the field of orthopedics, regenerative medicine has become an emerging practice that is offering relief for patients whose pain is caused by injuries, degeneration, or wear and tear of ligaments and tendons that support and stabilize joints. The goal of regenerative medicine is to stimulate the repair or replacement of damaged tissues through the augmentation of the body's own restorative processes.[13] In other words, these procedures aim to help facilitate a process that creates living and functional tissue where it has been damaged or compromised to help restore more normal function.

Regenerative procedures can be utilized for most joints in the body that may be causing pain, including, for example, spinal segments of the back or neck, sacroiliac joints, hips, and knees.

There are many types of regenerative musculoskeletal procedures, including needling tissues (also known as dry needling), injecting damaged tissue with whole blood, and injecting stem cells. The three most common forms include prolotherapy, platelet-rich plasma therapy, and stem cell therapy.

Originating in the 1930s, prolotherapy, also called sclerotherapy or now more commonly regenerative injection therapy, is the oldest and perhaps the most researched of these therapies. It involves injecting an irritant solution into a painful joint and its supporting ligaments and tendons. The idea is that joints that have lost stability due to repetitive stress or injuries can lose normal mechanics, degenerate, and cause pain, and that by injecting an irritant solution, usually a sterile dextrose (a type of sugar) solution, into the joint or where the connective tissues attach, a controlled, inflammatory response occurs that draws the body's normal healing process to the injected areas. With a series of repeated injections, this response stimulates the growth of new connective tissues that support the joint and within the joint, thereby helping reduce pain.

Prolotherapy has been used for low-back pain, headaches and neck pain, and wear-and-tear joint arthritis. It has also been used on joints that have suffered repetitive sprains. Research is still emerging, and therefore, prolotherapy is considered experimental by most insurance companies. As a result, it is not typically covered by insurance plans. However, more recent studies are showing promise for clinical outcomes and reinforce the proposed theory for how it works.

The most promising research involves osteoarthritis of the knee.[14] Research led by David Rabago at the University of Wisconsin compared results of patients who received prolotherapy injections with a dextrose solution, those who received a "sham" sterile saline injection, and those who received only home exercise treatments. After the initial injections, there was not a lot of difference between the subjects. However, as time progressed, those who received the series of dextrose solution injections reported significantly less pain and stiffness, with increased function, compared to those who received the saline injections and those who followed the home exercise protocol. These differences were noted even at week fifty-two of the study. Participants who received the injections reported high satisfaction results and felt the injections were safe and well tolerated. These results were similar to two random controlled trials[15] and a systematic review study of prolotherapy for osteoarthritis of the knee.[16]

Further research is ongoing to fully illuminate all the types of pain for which prolotherapy might be used. While the use of prolotherapy is supported in systematic reviews of literature for tendinopathies, knee and finger joint pain from wear-and-tear arthritis, and pelvic and spinal pain from ligament compromise, the jury is still out regarding its use for acute pain and myofascial pain.[17] A Cochrane review of the literature was less supportive of prolotherapy for chronic low-back pain, citing conflicting evidence between studies in which prolotherapy was offered alone and those in which it was used in combination with manipulation, exercises, and other treatment. In this review, those who received the additional modalities fared better than those who received prolotherapy alone.[18]

The use of platelet-rich plasma or stem cells in regenerative injection procedures has developed within the past thirty years. Both procedures are an expansion of the concept of prolotherapy, but they use different solutions and thus different mechanisms to stimulate the proliferation and regrowth of tissue. With platelet-rich plasma, blood is drawn from the patient receiving the procedure, the platelets and plasma are separated from whole blood through centrifuge, and then they are reinjected into the supporting structures of the patient's joint. Researchers state that healing is thought to be caused by the platelet-rich plasma's innate ability to draw cells into the area that foster regeneration of the same type of tissue that was compromised.[19]

Stem cell therapy uses the injection of stem cells typically derived from bone marrow, though cells obtained from adipose tissue (fat cells) or from the same individual can also be used. Stem cells are able to grow, develop, and replicate into many different types of cells based on local cell signaling pathways where they are placed.[20] In other words, it is thought that when injected into a tissue, they proliferate and take on the characteristics of the tissue, thus restoring normal mechanics and function to the affected joint.

Additional research is needed to evaluate how regenerative musculoskeletal injection procedures increase function, what mechanisms are employed in the healing process that is stimulated, and what biological markers could be used to verify those mechanisms or to support effectiveness.

How would you determine if regenerative musculoskeletal injection might work for you? The main thing is if you have pain to which you can directly point. This could be at the back of the neck, the base of the skull, the shoulder, the inner or outer elbow, the sides of the knee, the sacroiliac joint, or other common places where tissue injuries occur.

Typically, a series of injections would be needed for a full course of treatment for a specific pain condition. Be aware that the injections cause mild to moderate pain for a few days after the injection.[21] In the case of prolotherapy, this is because the injection is *meant* to cause inflammation as a way to initiate the body's healing processes. NSAIDs cannot be used to control this intended response, so typically acetaminophen is used for discomfort.

One of the main difficulties that faces the field of musculoskeletal regenerative medicine is a lack in standardization regarding the procedures and the methodology. So when selecting a physician to provide this therapy, ask where they received training and what credentials they have. The two main bodies that provide training at a national level are the Hackett Hemwall Patterson Foundation and the American Association of Orthopaedic Medicine. Other training programs are offered in the university setting, such as at the University of Wisconsin Prolotherapy and Education Lab. Once again, word of mouth in your area can sometimes be helpful, especially with specialized services like this. If people are getting good results, ask them about their experience and explore further.

Cannabinoid Medications

When discussing pain management, inevitably the use of marijuana to control pain comes up, though the discussions can be polarizing. Marijuana, also called cannabis (the scientific name), has been used for health conditions for centuries. Cannabinoids are natural or synthetic derivatives from the marijuana plant. There are passionate advocates and naysayers. Whenever I (Linda) blog on an update, I receive both criticism and praise, depending on the positions people take on this issue.

For the purposes of this book, it is not our intent to take a definitive stance on medical marijuana, as the data to date simply does not justify a solid position. We do, however, want to provide information concerning marijuana as a treatment for chronic pain. In the medical world, the effectiveness of a treatment is based on the evidence, not personal stories, testimonies, or legislative initiatives. While stories can be compelling, we have to follow the scientific evidence.

One of the problems surrounding the use of marijuana for pain management has been the difficulty conducting marijuana research in the US. It is our hope that high-quality research studies can be generated in order to develop guidelines for medical marijuana use in the near future.

In addition to the need for more studies, currently there are numerous inconsistencies between states for how medical marijuana is used.[22] At the time of this writing, medical marijuana is legal in thirty-two states and Washington, DC, but it is still illegal on the federal level. It is rated as a schedule 1 drug, meaning that it has high potential for abuse with "no currently accepted medical use."[23]

Marijuana is complex, containing four hundred compounds and approximately seventy cannabinoids other than the well-known tetrahydrocannabinol (THC). These compounds are not fully understood in terms of how they contribute to marijuana's effect.[24]

The compound cannabidiol (CBD) does not produce the high associated with THC because it does not affect the same brain receptors. It comes from the hemp plant, a cousin to the marijuana plant. It is usually extracted from the plant in oil or powder form and then mixed as a gel or cream that is rubbed on localized areas of pain. It comes in many forms with varying strengths and concentrations.

To date, there have been few clinical trials concerning the use of CBD for chronic pain. That said, some studies suggest that this compound was helpful with chronic inflammation and neuropathic pain in laboratory animals.[25] A 2018 report published in the *Cochrane Database of Systematic Reviews* looked at a variety of cannabis-based medicines and concluded that they may have some benefit for the treatment of chronic neuropathic pain.[26] However, large, well-designed clinical trials are lacking at the present time.

Concerns relating to CBD use center on the mild side effects of nausea, fatigue, skin irritations, and irritability. Of more concern are the potential for interactions with medications, a lack of regulation, the purity and content of CBD oils, and state laws that may prohibit CBD oil in a particular state. The substance does not currently have FDA approval, as it has the same classification as marijuana. While anecdotal data is mostly positive, there is still much to learn about CBD as related to chronic pain. You should discuss the legality and the use of CBD with your physician.

For medical marijuana, psychiatrists Deepak D'Souza and Mo-hini Ranganathan outline a number of concerns.[27] First, they note that studies involving individual cannabinoids such as THC and CBD cannot be extrapolated to general studies on marijuana. The composition of various cannabis preparations are varied, and there is little data on dosing smoked marijuana in terms of the medical conditions for which it is used.[28]

Second, there is not good data on the impact of repeated exposure to marijuana. Perhaps the greatest concern is that people may develop addiction, tolerance, and dependency, requiring dosage to be increased over time to be effective. At a recent academic conference, it was reported that 10 percent of users become addicted.[29] Exposing people to marijuana without conclusive evidence of its effectiveness for pain may increase the problem of abuse.

Another concern is that in some cases marijuana use can prompt psychotic disorders or exacerbate symptoms and relapse in some patients.[30] Because of this, people with schizophrenia, bipolar disorder, or substance abuse issues have contraindications for use.

Also, preclinical studies indicate that when adolescents are exposed to cannabinoids, they create long-lasting changes in the endocannabinoid systems and other neurotransmitter systems.[31] The endocannabinoid system is important in brain development and can impact a teen's emotional, cognitive, and behavioral development into adulthood. When any substance enters the body, the developing brain can be altered in ways that impact future health. Thus, the age of the person seeking medical marijuana treatment needs to be considered.

Finally, we don't know exactly how marijuana interacts with other drugs a person may be taking. One argument in favor of marijuana use is that it may decrease opioid use, but so far that conclusion is not supported.[32] Those who use marijuana because they have opioid use disorder don't reduce their use of opioids, and 39 percent of people who are longtime opioid users also use pot.[33]

The National Academies of Sciences, Engineering, and Medicine reviewed twenty-eight randomized studies. In their report, *The Health Effects of Cannabis and Cannabinoids*, they concluded that cannabinoids had a modest effect on adult chronic pain. Seventeen of the studies were related to neuropathic pain (nerve pain). In addition, cannabis helped with nausea and vomiting related to cancer chemotherapy, but there was little evidence to support its use for cancer pain.[34] And most of these studies did not compare cannabis to other ways to relieve pain.

The reviewers did note, "Thus, while the use of cannabis for the treatment of pain is supported by well-controlled clinical trials as reviewed above, very little is known about the efficacy, dose, routes of administration, or side effects of commonly used and commercially available cannabis products in the United States."[35] Donald Abrams, one of the reviewers and a professor of clinical medicine at the University of California, San Francisco, stated that there is a lack of evidence about the health effects of marijuana.[36]

Downsides to marijuana use include more car accidents, unintentional overdose injuries among children, increase in bronchitis when smoked, increase in schizophrenia and depression, low birth rates, and more. Marijuana use can also affect heart rate, blood pressure, and balance.[37]

At an academic conference, the following information was presented, which represents our current view on marijuana: "If the states' initiative to legalize medical marijuana is merely a veiled step toward allowing access to recreational marijuana, then the medical community should be left out of the process. Conversely, if the goal is to make marijuana available for medical purposes, then it is unclear why the approval process should be different from that for other medications."[38]

Clearly, this is a treatment for which more studies are needed. The jury is still out on the effectiveness and the cost-benefits in terms of the science.

Brain Stimulation Techniques (Nonsurgical)

In the search for noninvasive treatments for chronic pain, researchers have turned to a number of electrical brain stimulation techniques. Transcranial magnetic stimulation (TMS), a neuromodulation technique, has been used to stimulate nerve cells in the brain as a treatment for depression. Now it is being applied to pain in order to see if this is a viable noninvasive intervention. Five main types of treatments have emerged over the years: repetitive transcranial magnetic stimulation (rTMS), cranial electrotherapy stimulation (CES), transcranial direct current stimulation (tDCS), reduced impedance noninvasive cortical electrostimulation (RINCE), and transcranial random noise stimulation (tRNS).[39]

The technique that has been studied the most is rTMS. An electromagnetic field via a coil is generated by a machine and targeted directly to the brain. The idea is that the magnetic field modulates brain circuits and changes the brain. While the reasons this may reduce pain are not clearly understood, one thought is that malfunctioning connections between the motor circuits and sensory processing circuits are disrupted.[40]

Protocols for using rTMS vary, the frequency and duration of treatments are not standardized, and who would benefit the most from these treatments is still unknown. Multiple sessions are usually needed to reshape signaling in circuits involving chronic pain. At least this is the current thinking. Yet questions remain as to which specific brain area to target.

For a Cochrane report on the effectiveness of single doses of high-frequency rTMS on chronic pain,[41] reviewers looked at forty-two rTMS studies and determined that a small but consistent reduction in patient-reported pain was found as compared to sham controls. Mostly, the finding was related to chronic, intractable neuropathic pain. The studies were small and few, so no conclusions can be reached as to how effective rTMS is for chronic pain. But because it is a noninvasive procedure with few side effects (headaches, nausea, tingling, light-headedness, skin irritations, and on rare occasions seizures, mania, and hearing loss if the ears aren't protected during treatment), researchers are conducting studies to see if this is a pain management tool for the future. Under the section labeled "bottom line" of the Cochrane report is this sentence: "There is a lack of high-quality evidence to support or refute the effectiveness of non-invasive brain stimulation techniques for chronic pain."[42] Bottom, bottom line: The jury is still out.

Overall, more studies are needed to determine the effectiveness of complementary and alternative approaches to pain management. Public opinion and the passion of advocacy groups can be strong, but follow the science and consult a physician to determine the best approaches to help you live beyond pain.

PART 3

HOPE *and* RESILIENCE

21

Develop a Positive Mind-Set

Reflect upon your present blessings—of which every man
has many—not on your past misfortunes, of which all men
have some.

Charles Dickens

Laura is a young woman who suffers from chronic back pain. She
constantly says things like "There is too much wear and tear on
this broken body" or "I feel like I am sixty years old" when she feels
pain. Multiple times a day she makes negative comments about her
pain and associates her pain with "broken, old, and wear and tear."

What Laura doesn't realize is that during this process, her brain
is creating a folder named "Back Pain" that is filtering her words. In
the folder is a stored document called "Broken," another document
called "Wear and Tear," and another called "Old." The more she
makes negative comments about her back pain, the more her brain
keeps creating documents and saving them. The folder is becoming full of negative associations. When she has a pain incident,
the folder pulls up the documents to help her interpret what she
is feeling. Messages such as broken, old, and wear and tear are

retrieved and she feels worse. Then she says, "It's no use. I will be living with this pain the rest of my life." Laura has used her words to create a negative mind-set toward her pain.

What is going on? The billions of neurons in the brain form connections with other neurons to send signals in the brain. As a group of neurons grows, so does its ability to send messages throughout the brain. In that process, the nervous system creates memories or what are called neurosignatures or neurotags. A neurotag is simply a pattern of neuron activation that creates outputs in the brain. Those outputs can be perception, thought, movement, or immune responses.[1] This is how the brain remembers what it learns.

You may have heard the saying "Neurons that fire together, wire together." Neurons become activated (fire) and link together (wire) to interpret a single input from a neurotag and can trigger memory. Neurotags form and strengthen through repetition and in other ways. Eventually, neurons can fire at just the thought of something.

Pain is an output of a physical linking of neurotags at a particular time. We are not conscious of this process, but we have a very personalized neurosignature for pain.[2] Thoughts and emotions are connected to neurotag networks and can become sensitized and remembered. For example, a neurotag for "back pain" may be associated with one called "slipped disc." When the slipped disc neurotag is activated, it is likely that the back pain neurotag will also be activated. Thus, thinking about a slipped disc can activate pain.

According to pain specialist G. Lorimer Moseley, we can create and modify our neurotags in many ways.[3] Moving in new ways to stimulate the nervous system is one example. We can also change our pain associations by being positive about pain and not creating negative associations.

Remember Carol Dweck's concept of the growth mind-set discussed in chapter 12? When you have a growth mind-set, you can grow, overcome adversity, and change your pain. Pain doesn't have to define you. It's a problem to be faced. As you change your thoughts and behaviors, you change your brain. With a growth mind-set, you can live beyond pain. Mind-set matters when dealing with chronic pain and makes a difference in how you feel. It is how you create a positive neurosignature.

If you expect to feel worse, to not get better, to have your life ruined by pain, you have a negative (fixed) mind-set that will keep you stuck. Such expectations prime your nervous system for more pain. They will also undermine your recovery and enhance your pain.

Instead, you want to prime your brain for pain relief. For example, if you are thinking, *I can't get off these opioids or the pain will be unbearable*, you are priming your brain for more pain. However, if you think, *I can get off these opioids. I will feel bad for a while, but then I will feel better*, you are priming your brain for pain relief. Positive expectations will push you forward to grow. They will erase those old documents in the folder and replace them with new ones.

If you refuse to give in to pain and fight back with all the tools you have learned so far, you will create a growth mind-set. Maybe you haven't solved all your issues yet, but you are working on them one by one—remembering the importance of marginal gains. The goal is to thrive, not simply survive, so here are a few more ways to develop a positive mind-set while dealing with pain.

Use Positive Affirmations

It is important to remind yourself daily that you are not your pain. Don't allow pain to take over your life and dominate your thoughts. If you think only negative thoughts, you will see only the negative. Here are a few positive affirmations to help you create a more positive approach to pain:

Pain is temporary.
Pain is not in charge of my life.

Pain will not kill me.

Pain tests my character, but it won't win.

This, too, shall pass.

Pain does not keep me from being me.

God has given me what I need to deal with pain today.

I am strong enough to handle this pain.

I am not a victim of my pain.

Begin your day with a positive affirmation: "Today I will manage my pain." Think about the things in your life that are positive and good. This is an intentional process of focusing your mind on a positive aspect of your life when you start your day. For example, "I am blessed to live in a place where I can look out my window and see mountains" or, "There is beauty all around me if I look for it." By saying positive affirmations, you are training your brain to focus on things of joy, positive experiences, the goodness of God, daily blessings, and more. Every day you can find positive things to focus on if you look. Using positive affirmations is a type of pain relief. It is powerful. It won't make pain disappear, but it will help your experience of pain.

Practice Gratitude

You might be thinking, *I am in pain. Why should I be grateful?* Because there are so many other parts of your life—moments and experiences—that are positive. Gratitude is a state of thankfulness and appreciation. It is an attitude, something most of us have to cultivate because it is easy to focus on negatives. Practicing gratitude doesn't mean you ignore your pain. Rather, you choose not to let it define you or your day.

When we express gratitude, it makes us feel good. It creates positive emotions and even feelings of happiness. One reason for this is that expressing gratitude can release the bonding hormone oxytocin.[4] This physiological release decreases the release of stress hormones, such as cortisol, and promotes health. The science of gratitude is linked to a host of health benefits. Gratitude has been shown to lower blood pressure and boost the immune system related to cardiac health, to name just a few.[5]

Practicing gratitude has also been linked to better sleep.[6] Try being grateful and focus on the blessings of the day before you put your head on the pillow. Count your blessings before you go to sleep. Doing so relaxes you and puts you in a positive frame of mind. The more you focus on the positives of your day, the less worry and negativity will fill your mind. Gratitude can also decrease feelings of depression and anxiety.[7] Focusing on what you appreciate about others and about your life puts you in a positive state of mind and helps you fall asleep.

To better illustrate the effects of gratitude, consider a study conducted by researchers Robert Emmons and Michael McCullough, who wanted to see if gratitude would have an effect on well-being. They compared three groups of people: those in one group kept a gratitude journal, those in a second group focused on negative life events (or what they called hassles), and those in a third group focused on neutral events. What they discovered was that the people in the gratitude-focused group felt better about their lives, were more optimistic, and reported fewer physical complaints. In addition, the gratitude group had improvement in sleep in that they got more hours of sleep at night. Even the spouses of the people in the gratitude group noticed a positive change.[8]

You don't have to keep a gratitude journal, but some people find that a journal helps them focus. And the benefit of a journal is that on a bad pain day, you can go back and read an entry that will remind you of your blessings. You are not denying your pain but rather choosing to focus on things in your day that are positive—the smile of your child, the beauty of the landscape, the help of a stranger, the comforting words of your spouse. The change in focus away from the pain helps you feel better.

An easy way to begin practicing gratitude is to do so at the beginning and the end of every day. Think of three things you can count as blessings. At first, doing this might be difficult simply because you are not used to this focus. But over time, it will be easier because you will be more tuned in to finding the positives. In fact, a focus on gratitude can be learned.

Pain patient Renee will tell you that her first thought every day when she awakened was, *Okay, here we go again. I am already in pain. How is this day going to go? I'd rather stay in bed.* Basically, Renee started her day with a sense of dread and believed she was caught in a repeating cycle of pain she could not escape. As a result, she grew more negative and isolated. She did not want to engage with people because she knew she would have to cut the time short due to pain.

Renee decided to take on the gratitude challenge. Some days were easier than others when it came to counting blessings. But she hung in there and was determined to make a change in this area. Eventually, she concluded that there is always something to be grateful for—no matter how small. She could find something good in every day. She is still living with chronic pain due to fibromyalgia, but she finds moments in her day for which to be grateful. It has made a difference in her outlook on life.

And then there is Christy, my (Linda's) former hairdresser, who experienced a horrific trauma by surviving a house fire. She was burned on her arms, back, and hands, requiring grafts. Christy was in excruciating pain and had to fight back to recover and heal for over two years. After the trauma, she wanted to regain some sense of normalcy in her life. As her burns began to heal, she was able to do hair again. This was quite remarkable given that the burns on her arms and hands were severe and the doctors were uncertain whether she would regain enough feeling to do it. But Christy is a fighter and refused to give in to "can't." When she did my hair, she often talked about the parts of her experience that involved gratitude: she didn't die in the fire, her face was not badly burned, her children were safe, and she could still use her hands. Every time we talked, her conversation was filled with gratitude for the help of so many people. I am convinced that her attitude of thankfulness and gratitude was a part of her healing. Gratitude and well-being are related.[9]

To help you get started practicing gratitude, here are ten ideas from people in pain who know the importance of gratitude in terms of keeping their outlook positive:

1. Start noticing any small thing that brings you pleasure or joy. Don't negate anything in the process. Something as inconsequential as light traffic on the way home from work can be noticed.

2. Start a gratitude challenge with a friend or family member. If you want to improve good feelings toward a partner, this can help.

3. Use mindfulness and make a blessing the focus.

4. Journal your gratitude moments and read through them regularly to remind you of your many blessings.

5. Volunteer your time. One of the many benefits of volunteering is that gratitude is contagious. People thank you, and you feel grateful to them.

6. Write thank-you letters to people, especially those who have contributed to your life. If you aren't a letter writer, send a text. A quick message can boost your mood and the mood of others.

7. Set a goal to express gratitude to one or two people a day. They could be a coworker, a boss, a neighbor, a family member—anyone is fair game.

8. Make a gratitude jar and have anyone who lives with you contribute slips of paper to the jar. Periodically, pull out the slips of paper and read them. This is an exercise often done at Thanksgiving, but it can be done all year round.

If it is done in a family setting, children learn to focus on blessings too.

9. Look for someone who rarely gets a thank-you and target that person for gratitude (e.g., the janitor in your building, the fast-food server, the complaints person at a business, etc.).

10. Smile and disrupt the flow of negativity. Flashing a smile can be a visual reminder that there is much to be happy about in life despite your challenges.

These small changes—marginal gains—can change your mind-set and help with pain. Give thanks with a grateful heart. It's good medicine for the soul.

Learn to Forgive

When you live with pain, it is tempting to listen to that small voice whispering in your ear, "Why you? This isn't fair. You don't deserve this. People are insensitive and indifferent. They don't understand." The result of such thoughts can be resentment and even bitterness. Both can lead to self-pity and misery. A way to protect yourself is to make forgiveness a part of a positive mind-set.

People who treat chronic pain report that some patients have trouble forgiving people whom they feel have offended them in some way.[10] And when unforgiveness is present, chronic pain goes up. Unforgiveness has an impact on the physical body via the nervous and endocrine systems. The distress associated with unforgiveness can be transformed into pain. But forgiveness can promote health. [11]

Consider Mandy's story. For years, she sat alone in her home, ruminating on all the wrongs that had been committed against her. She was so miserable that she agreed to see a pain psychologist. The anger and resentment she felt toward people who had let her down or rejected her were significant.

The psychologist had Mandy list all the offenses and wrongs she felt. The list was long. One by one, Mandy went through her list and made a decision to forgive each person who had wounded her. There was her ex-husband, who had been unfaithful; a family member who had accused her of being self-centered; a friend who had abandoned her due to pain interfering with plans; a doctor who had been insensitive to her plight; and so on.

As Mandy worked through her list and dealt with the bitterness that had developed, she noticed less pain daily. Unforgiveness had changed her in ways she hadn't noticed. It had cost her time, energy, and relationships. When Mandy reverted in her thinking and focused on injustices, she noticed an increase in her pain level. The contrast was so striking that she canceled an upcoming elective surgery for pain relief because of the differences she felt in her physical body when she focused on forgiveness. In Mandy's case, unforgiveness played a major role in increasing her pain. Forgiveness was a gift she gave herself. It freed her from bitterness and resentment—and pain.

Steven Hayes, the founder of acceptance and commitment therapy, says this about holding on to unforgiveness: "Unforgiveness is like being on a giant hook. Next to you on the hook is the person who has hurt you. The hook is extremely painful. Wherever you go, so does the hook and so does the offender. The only way you can get off the hook is if you allow the offender off first."[12] You can make the choice to get off the hook.

One of the reasons people struggle with forgiveness is because they misunderstand it. They think it means accepting what the person did or convincing themselves that what happened wasn't hurtful. But that is not the case. It is about making a decision not to let what happened lead to bitterness. While we don't have control over many things that happen to us, we do have control over our reactions. Forgiveness is an action within our control.

It is also a process. Emotions often need to catch up to the decision to forgive. It takes time to emotionally work through an offense. Forgiveness researchers Robert Enright and Richard Fitzgibbons have outlined four stages of the forgiveness process.[13]

First is the uncovering stage. You think about what happened, gather information, and determine how what happened affected you. Basically, who did what to whom. During this stage, it helps to ask questions such as, How is unforgiveness affecting me? How much space is unforgiveness occupying in my life? Am I avoiding a necessary part of my healing?

Next is the decision phase. You make a decision to forgive, recognizing that not doing so will cost you more pain. What has been stopping you from letting go? What has blocked you from choosing to forgive?

The third phase is the working phase. You do the work of forgiveness, dealing with your emotional reactions, trying to extend empathy and compassion toward others, and moving through difficult feelings. This part of forgiveness cannot be rushed or demanded. It is the hardest part of the process because you can make a decision to forgive without working through the related emotions. Overcoming negative feelings changes you in terms of motivation, thoughts, and eventually behavior. When you truly work through the emotional process of forgiveness, you begin to consider the other person and feel empathy.

Finally, during the deepening phase, you feel release and give meaning to the importance of forgiveness and confront suffering. When forgiveness is worked through on a deep level, it promotes health. It combats stress, hostility, and rumination.

Forgiveness doesn't mean you minimize the hurt you felt when offended or treated poorly. It doesn't excuse or justify behavior. It actually does the opposite. It acknowledges that you have suffered. In spite of that, you are choosing to forgive. You are no longer allowing the person to have power over you. You are giving up your right to resentment or to seek revenge. Forgiveness doesn't make the other person right, but it can set you free.

Forgiveness is also not the same as reconciliation. It has been said that forgiveness is a one-way street, but reconciliation is a two-way street. Reconciliation requires the cooperation of both parties. It requires the willingness of both parties to make things right. Thus, forgiving someone doesn't automatically mean there is a reestablished trust. Forgiveness is a single act, one you can do regardless of whether or not the other person cooperates. But it does require an acceptance of what happened and a recognition of how you have been affected. You may not forget a wrong that was done to you, but you can forgive the wrong and move forward regardless of the action of the other person.

In a psychological sense, forgiveness is the process of letting go and working through the emotions associated with the process. It is a recognition that you have a personal responsibility to do something that can aid your well-being. It can help you heal as well as help others.[14]

It is interesting that forgiveness is a part of the belief system of five major religions in the world (Christianity, Islam, Judaism, Buddhism, and Hinduism). In Christianity, forgiveness is a central tenet that was exercised by Christ toward his executioners and the religious leaders. It is also a command given to his followers. As we have been forgiven, we are to forgive others.

To develop a positive mind-set, use positive affirmations, practice gratitude, and learn to forgive. Such actions involve areas of your life over which you can exercise control and can lead to positive emotions and attitudes that can help you live beyond pain.

22

Make Meaning out of Pain and Suffering

Everywhere a greater joy is preceded by a greater suffering.

St. Augustine

Unfortunately, pain and suffering are a part of our lives, and we all encounter our share of both in a lifetime. Because of this reality, we have included a chapter on the meaning of pain and suffering from a spiritual perspective. The spiritual side of pain and suffering has to be reckoned with if you want to deal with pain in a holistic way. And the science literature shows that both spirituality and religion influence pain in positive ways.[1] We are firm believers that to effectively deal with pain, you have to find a way to make meaning out of your pain. Otherwise, it is too easy to sink into despair.

Joni Eareckson Tada is no stranger to chronic pain. She has lived all her adult life as a quadriplegic due to a diving accident at the age of seventeen. Her ability to cope with her condition and pain comes from a deep spiritual place. She says, "Pain and chronic illness can make you question God and His power. Because we know God holds the keys of the universe, we also know He sees and governs everything that happens on earth."[2] Tada reminds us that it is normal to question God and to be fearful in times of pain, but we can't allow fear or doubt to dictate our lives. If we do, our lives will be miserable.

When my (Linda's) brother was killed years ago, I was desperate to understand why—why would a loving God allow such a painful outcome? It didn't fit into my way of thinking about God. I had been raised in the church, but I had never been tested by such a personally painful event. This circumstance that caused great family suffering pushed me to search for answers. Could I really trust God to be loving when such pain occurred? Any number of you could ask the same question. Why am I in pain, disabled, dealing with cancer or disease? Why doesn't the pain stop? Why does a good God allow suffering?

We aren't the first or the last people to struggle with these types of questions. Throughout the ages, people of all kinds have grappled with why a good and loving God allows suffering. We felt it important to offer some thoughts and provide a way to think about suffering that will hopefully transform your pain into something meaningful. We are not theologians but rather practitioners who desire to help people come to terms with their pain. We do, however, believe in the basic tenets of the Christian faith. If this is not your perspective, we encourage you to find meaning in your pain in ways that are consistent with your beliefs in order to prevent despair. We know through research and years of clinical experience that faith helps people in pain.

We have already established that how we think about pain and suffering matters because our beliefs generate our thoughts, impact our emotions, and direct our behaviors. Based on our beliefs, we can end up angry and bitter, feeling abandoned and not cared about by anyone. Or we can find peace, trust, and acceptance.

Our responses to pain and suffering matter, and those responses are generated by our beliefs.

The Question of Suffering

There are no easy answers to the question of suffering. Sometimes there are no answers at all. We don't know the mind of God and do not have his understanding. Still, we can learn much about pain and suffering from those who have gone before us who have been tried and tested. But each person must come to terms with what it means when they suffer.

Holly grew up in the church, but recently she found herself doubting her faith. Her health had taken a downward turn, and she was racked with pain almost daily. The platitudes from church members, "Bad things happen to good people," "God is in control," "God won't give you more than you can handle," didn't help or bring her closer to God. The borrowed faith of her parents was not working. It was time to make faith her own. Until now, nothing had really challenged her to question God or wonder if he was working in her life. Holly decided to employ a spiritual formation coach who understood the mind, body, and spirit connection for healing.

Holly took time to do abiding prayer in which she allowed God to lead her to the awareness of his presence. She used religious images to help focus her mind on God. As Holly sat in silence and meditated on biblical phrases, she rested in God's presence. She did this with no agenda but to listen to God. Meditation and solitude were ways to explore her heart. The more she meditated on God and his Word, the more she realized her circumstances did not determine God's great love for her. Then her spiritual coach recommended a twenty-four-hour fast from food and all media. During that time, Holly was astounded at how much she depended on media and how little she depended on God. These spiritual disciplines helped her develop a new habit of turning to God to deepen her attachment to him.

Holly and her coach decided to evaluate Holly's progress by asking two questions. The first was, Do I love God more today than I did before? Holly felt she was deepening her attachment to God through her time with him. As she sat in his presence and quieted herself, she was refreshed by God's love.

But the second question was much more challenging. It had to do with her obedience. How well does my life line up with what I believe? The obstacles to her growth included busyness, distraction from entertainment, and her tendency to be self-centered. If she was honest, there was still too much *self* in her life that was not focusing on love and compassion for others.

So daily she exposed herself to Scripture and chose one command to follow (e.g., the command to bless God at all times). She spent twenty minutes a day opening her heart in prayer and evaluating her life choices. She asked the question, What is blocking me from doing the things that would help my life flourish?

As Holly engaged with God, worry was replaced with trust. Through this process, her faith roots deepened and she found contentment. Even with the pain, she realized she could be grateful and trust God. Her faith was becoming her own, and it was transforming her life.

A Spiritual Lens on Suffering

Holly's wrestling with pain involved a spiritual path, one that led her to a way to think about and respond to pain. She chose to look at pain through a spiritual lens and to see God's presence in her life. You can do the same.

God doesn't downplay the suffering we face. He doesn't tell us not to hurt or minimize our pain. The prophet Isaiah tells us that God is acquainted with our grief (Isa. 53:3). The promise is that he is present and will walk with us through pain and suffering. When we hurt, God is with us.

Bestselling author Philip Yancey asks the question, Where is God when it hurts? in his book by the same title. His answer: God is in us. He hasn't abandoned us, hasn't forgotten about us, and isn't reveling in our suffering. He abides in us, promising his peace and even joy despite our circumstances.[3] Peter Kreeft, in his book *Making Sense Out of Suffering*, comes to the same conclusion. God gave us himself. And while it may not seem as if God is better than any pill or advice we can offer, he has the power to heal, to stop anxiety, to trade hope for despair, and to bring joy out of sorrow.[4]

Still, why doesn't God stop suffering? After all, he hates to see his creation suffer. Some would assert that pain and suffering are a part of free will. God created humans with free will so that we could choose whether to love him. If we did not have the ability to choose good over evil or to choose God no matter what, we would be robots and our love for God would be meaningless. But with free will came the potential for pain and suffering. We are tarnished by sin, and pain and suffering are a part of the fallen human condition.

Whatever the reason, all people, religious and nonreligious, recognize that pain and suffering exist. However, God can use pain to bring about good. Pain draws us close to him, often makes us desperate for him, and reminds us of our weakness and dependence on him. Author C. S. Lewis says, "God whispers in our pleasure, speaks in our conscience, but shouts in our pain."[5] For those of you in pain, there is a lot of shouting going on. But if we listen, pain can be transformed and bring humility, trust, faith, and even gratitude into our lives. If we accept pain as a part of our fallen state, we can pray for it to be redeemed.

English writer Dorothy Sayers provides more perspective on God and suffering when she writes:

> For whatever reason God chose to make people as they are—limited and suffering and subject to sorrow and death—He had the honesty

and courage to take His own medicine. Whatever game He is playing with His creation, He has kept His own rules and played fair. He can exact nothing from us that He has not exacted from Himself. He has Himself gone through the whole human experience, from the trivial irritations of family life and the cramping restrictions of hard work and lack of money to the worst horrors of pain and humiliation, defeat, despair, and death. When He was man, He played the man. He was born in poverty and died in disgrace and thought it was all worthwhile.[6]

God knows our pain and is straight with us. He didn't lie and try to sell us a bill of goods. He didn't campaign on the slogan "Join with me and you will have a pain-free life." No, he informed us that on this side of eternity there will be pain and suffering. Pastor and apologist Tim Keller reminds us that pain and suffering exist not because God doesn't love us. If he didn't love us, he would not have gone to the cross. Thus, pain and suffering do not discount a loving God. Our loving God takes our suffering seriously, and through his resurrection, he gives us a glimpse of what is to come: a reversal of pain and death.[7]

If we begin with the premise that God is good and loving, then this belief will inform our thoughts, emotions, and behaviors. God is not a meanie, allowing things to happen in our lives for no redemptive purpose. It took me (Linda) awhile to believe this in my own life because I didn't study the character of God. I simply went by how I felt (known as emotional reasoning). I was mad at God when I felt pain. I wanted to think God was angry and punishing my family, but I could find no proof of this in Scripture or in his actions with his people.

When we are in pain, it is easy to blame God or believe untrue things. Sometimes we falsely believe pain is punishment, but having pain doesn't mean we did something wrong. The book of Job proves this. The book begins with an assertion that Job was a righteous man. Suffering did not come his way because of his sin or because he brought it on. In Job's case, suffering was a test. He had no idea why he suffered, and he never received an answer. Regardless, he made the decision to trust God in the middle of his pain, and God redeemed his life after repeated loss.

Sometimes suffering is a part of living in a diseased and fallen world. The rain of pain falls on the just and the unjust. Christians are not exempt from the natural causes of pain, the results of bad habits, or the aging process of the body.

We must be careful not to judge why someone goes through pain and suffering. Sometimes it is self-inflicted; other times it is not. Only God knows the reason for the struggle. What we do know is that our response to suffering is within our control. Psychologist Viktor Frankl, a survivor of a Nazi concentration camp, reminds us that we have the freedom to choose our attitudes in the middle of difficulty.[8] Frankl's life is an example of suffering that was delivered to him by the hands of evil men in powerful ways but also a witness that God is more powerful. Through his faith, he chose not to allow bitterness and despair to overtake him in the worst of circumstances but rather to search for meaning in the pain.

Suffering Creates a New You

Job's response to suffering brought him to a new relationship with God. Before his suffering, Job knew about God, but through his struggles, he encountered God and trusted him. At the end of his suffering process, Job realized that knowing God was better than an answer as to why he had suffered.

We may not like the process, but suffering is often used to refine us. Suffering can grow our faith if we approach it in an honest way. When we suffer, there can be a deepening in our walk and a new intimacy with God. When we suffer, there seems to be an opening of our souls and a cry for God's help in our lives. Like Job, we tend to experience God at a deeper level. Blaise Pascal chose to see his suffering as a way to grow his patience, take care of his health to better serve God, and focus more on his faith.[9] There are times when God allows suffering for a greater purpose to be accomplished in us and even in others. Our response is what we control.

Journalist Malcolm Muggeridge also referenced the importance of suffering in his own life, reflecting on how affliction made him grow and how suffering enlightened his life experience. Suffering and affliction, not success or happiness, taught him the most important things about life. Through his suffering, he was able to count it all joy, knowing that the trying of his faith brought perseverance and patience.[10]

Suffering, in the end, can create a better you. It often reveals the state of our hearts and can increase our faith. It has a way of bringing our strengths and weaknesses to the surface. God often purifies and refines us through suffering. Pain can produce growth and maturity in our faith walk if we trust God even when it hurts. Those difficult moments of darkness can lead us to depend on God's power, not our own.

We can begin to understand God's love through our own parenting experiences. There are times when our children are stubborn, even disobedient, and need to feel the pain of their choices. Other times they face hardship and difficulty we can't fix for them. I (Linda) remember one day when my son was in fourth grade and really struggling with a particular issue. I so badly wanted to intervene and make it better. But my son's very wise and experienced teacher told me to let him handle it. God was preparing in him a capacity for compassion for others in a way I could not. As loving parents, we find it difficult to watch our children struggle, but we know that the learning is in the struggle and the struggle is refining their character. During difficult times, we offer our presence and our love, but they have to work through the struggles needed to build their character and faith. As a good Father, God does the same. He always knows what is best for us. And he grieves with us when we are in pain and offers his presence.

So perhaps a good question to ask is, What does God desire from me during pain and suffering? Is it trust? Is he working all things for my good, a good I perhaps cannot see? If we see suffering as a refining fire, we can rejoice in our suffering. Why? Because suffering produces perseverance and perseverance produces character and character produces hope (Rom. 5:3–4).

Hang On to Hope

When there is healing, Swiss physician Paul Tournier frames it as a symbol of God's redemptive grace.[11] It is a reminder to us that God wins over death and disease. During his time on earth, Jesus healed people. He did it when people appealed to him in faith in order to evidence his power. Appeal to God during times of pain. Ask for healing. In faith, believe. All healing comes from God, whether by the hand of a doctor or a therapist or supernaturally. God intervenes in our brokenness, postponing the inevitability of death and showing his power. Healing is a sign of God's mercy.

But if healing does not come, hang on to hope. It may be difficult to hang on to hope in the face of suffering, but the only alternative is despair. Choose hope in order to make meaning out of suffering. God gave us his presence so that we can endure all things. He provides us with hope and a future.

Be reassured that tears are not a sign of weakness. God is okay with our struggle to trust him, but when we do, the change is transformative. We mourn our losses and cry out to God in times of pain. He who is acquainted with our grief and sorrow can handle it. Lament is prevalent in the Christian Bible. Psalm 13:1–2 is often the cry of the person in pain: "How long, Lord? Will you forget me forever? How long will you hide your face from me? How long must I wrestle with my thoughts and day after day have sorrow in my heart?" The psalmist concludes that he is not forgotten and that his suffering matters to God. God will sustain him.

Our options are to believe that God doesn't care about our suffering, that he doesn't exist at all, or that we truly do not understand his ways because they are higher than ours. We choose the latter. Don't turn up the volume on pain by allowing despair. Believe his goodness will sustain you. Use all the means we have suggested in this book to make pain less intrusive, more bearable, and perhaps even go away. But through the process, continue to ask, What can I learn from pain? What can God accomplish with me during this time? Can there be purpose in my pain?

Throughout this book, we have tried to convey that we are listening to those of you in pain. But more important for you to know is that God is listening. He wants to meet you where you are. You can experience his joy and peace in the middle of suffering. He will shape you more in his image. One day all pain will be gone. In the meantime, fight the good fight, pray for strength, hold on to hope, and do what you can to live beyond your pain and make meaning out of suffering.

23

Create a Personal Pain Plan

Hope begins in the dark, the stubborn hope that if you just
show up and try to do the right thing, the dawn will come.
You wait and watch and work; you don't give up.

Anne Lamott

We have discussed many areas of change that can add up to big
differences in terms of pain. Using the concept of marginal gains,
it is time to put it all together and develop a plan for your life.

Make Goals

A recent patient of mine (James's) is an avid runner. She used to
run half marathons, but because of her pain and some lingering
challenges with her gait, she hadn't been able to run for over three
years. I evaluated her, and we outlined a treatment plan together.
Then I asked her if she had any pictures of herself from any of
the running events she used to so deeply enjoy. She said she did. I
encouraged her to get them out and hang them up. I wanted her to

see them and for her to have a daily reminder of what she wanted back in her life. I wanted them to inspire her, to reorient her focus.

Just like an athlete training for an event, you are training for life and making changes that will make a difference. Setting goals is important because doing so forces you to stop and think about how you would like your life to be. This is powerful. Just having your thoughts on paper is a marginal gain. And when you begin to work toward the goals you have set, doing so diverts your focus from what is painful to what is possible.

So decide on your goals. Do you want to decrease pain intensity, reduce pain complaints, improve the quality of your life and functioning, and/or work on the physical, psychological, and social changes that could improve your pain? Do you want to play with your grandchildren again, take walks in the park, go hiking, or simply be able to navigate your daily life more independently?

Writing out your goals will help you evaluate your progress. The best approach is to break down your goals into small steps so you can monitor success along the way.

When you choose a goal, make sure it is specific in terms of behavior, is measurable, involves action, and is realistic and time specific. Once you have your goals, begin to develop a self-care plan that may also include professional care.

After reading all the factors involved with pain, you may feel a bit overwhelmed as to where to begin to make changes. But start *somewhere*. We encourage you to start small but not think of a small change as a small thing. Celebrate your achievements and even your partial victories, because success breeds success, and success builds momentum.

Following is a summary of all the areas discussed in which you can make a difference and begin to steer a course for change. Use the concept of marginal gains to improve one or two areas of your life, and then add more to build on your success. The point is to take charge when and where you can and to live your life to the fullest. You are here for a reason and have a purpose to fulfill.

Take Inventory

Loss of control	List ways to take back control.
Loss of enjoyment	List ways to create enjoyment.
Loss of work and passion	Create a financial plan to rebuild finances. Re-evaluate work and passion and determine a new normal.
Loss of identity	List ways to define yourself apart from your pain. I am _____.
Loss of function	Make a realistic appraisal of things you can do and goals for moving forward.
Loss of relationships	Talk to family and friends about the way pain can be less central and interfere less in your relationships. See a therapist if needed.
Loss of intimacy	Discuss with your partner how pain has affected your intimacy. See a therapist if needed.
Loss of dreams and expectations	Reassess your life story and establish new dreams and expectations.
Loss of hope	Hold on to hope through inspirational stories, people who have met challenges, and people who will lift you up. Find images, pictures, and quotes that will encourage you.

Traditional Approaches to Pain Management

When considering traditional approaches to pain management, discuss the following questions with a doctor:

- Are there long-term consequences to taking this medication?
- How do I store medications safely?
- What are the risks or side effects? What do I need to monitor?
- Are the benefits worth the side effects I might experience?

- If I want to stop taking a medication, is it safe to do so?
- How do you define treatment success?
- Is there anything else I can try? What else might work?

Change Your Structure

If your pain is related to structural issues, consider manipulation to correct the problems and alleviate your pain. Ask a physician or potential provider these questions:

- What are the risks?
- What are the alternatives?
- How do you define successful treatment?
- What should I expect, and when should I expect improvement?
- Will I be sore? What if the treatment causes more pain?

Change Your Beliefs

Assess your pain beliefs. Work to change negative beliefs to more hopeful and positive beliefs.

Write down your beliefs and identify negative beliefs that could be making you feel worse and increasing your pain. Challenge those beliefs. See chapter 12 for examples of negative beliefs and how to reframe them.

Change Your Thoughts

Remember that negative thoughts lead to negative feelings and behaviors, so challenge those negative thoughts and replace them with more positive ones. Assess your thinking and rate the frequency of your pain-related thoughts. See how much you ruminate on, magnify, and feel helpless about your pain. See chapter 13 for ways to identify and change catastrophic thinking.

Change Your Emotions

Are the following emotions contributing to your pain? If you need help regulating these emotions, see a therapist as an additional way to turn down the volume on pain.

- Fear: Name your fear and how it plays into avoidance.
- Anger: Is anger causing bitterness in your life?
- Depression: If your emotions have led to depression, make a plan to see a therapist and consider taking medication if that would help.

Change Your Relationships

As difficult as it might be, talk to your friends and family about how pain is impacting your relationships. Then make a few changes in the way you interact with those you care about:

- Focus your conversations less on pain and more on other parts of your life.
- Don't allow others to do for you when you can do for yourself.
- If you have children, explain to them what you can and cannot do, but find ways to involve yourself in their activities.
- Communicate your needs directly.
- Consider the type of work you can do regardless of pain.
- Stay connected to those you love and care about—do not isolate.
- Continue to grow from setbacks, be flexible, and don't give up.

- Talk with your intimate partner as to how pain can be lessened during sexual activity.

Change Your Stress

Which of the following techniques might you use to reduce stress:

- Distraction
- Relaxation methods
- Biofeedback
- Hypnosis
- Mindfulness

Change Your Lifestyle

Which of the following might help you reduce your pain:

- Avoiding alcohol
- Avoiding smoking
- Maintaining a healthy weight
- Keeping your body hydrated by drinking half your weight in ounces of water each day
- Eating an anti-inflammatory diet
- Getting an adequate amount of sleep

The Importance of Exercise and Movement

Because exercise and movement are so important to any pain plan, think of ways to incorporate both in your daily life:

- Choose low- to moderate-intensity ways to exercise (e.g., yoga, tai chi, Pilates)
- Increase daily movement

When You Need More Help

If you feel stuck and think therapy might help, consider the following types of therapies:

- Acceptance and commitment therapy
- Cognitive behavioral therapy
- Mindfulness-based stress reduction

Complementary and Alternative Approaches to Pain Management

Always check with your health care provider before you decide to use these approaches. Make sure the provider is someone who is experienced and well-trained:

- Acupuncture
- Regenerative medicine
- Cannabinoid medications
- Brain stimulation techniques

Develop a Positive Mind-Set

Thinking positively can go a long way toward moderating pain. Here are some ways you can develop a positive mind-set:

- Use positive affirmations
- Practice gratitude
- Learn to forgive

Make Meaning Out of Pain and Suffering

What are some ways you can hold on to hope and find meaning in your pain? Journal your thoughts. Talk to others who have suffered and experienced pain. Use your faith as a resource for resiliency and hope.

Epilogue

Never Give Up

When the unthinkable happens, the lighthouse is hope. Once we choose hope, everything is possible.

Christopher Reeve

Our message is one of hope. It's optimistic. You can build a better life and be a better you. Remain hopeful for a better tomorrow. Never give up on doing your part to improve your health and pain. Use everything you can to move through pain.

There are so many stories of people who refused to give up and give in to difficult life circumstances. They are overcomers and inspire us all to live with difficulty. Here is one of our favorites. It involves an Italian immigrant family who refused a negative report. They chose hope and developed resilience. Let their story inspire you to live beyond pain.

Mario "Motts" Tonelli was born to Italian immigrant parents and lived on the North Side of Chicago. Like most boys his age, he loved to play and run through the streets of his Chicago neighborhood with friends. On one of those days, a friend accidently knocked over a burning garbage barrel. It fell on six-year-old Mario.

The trash incinerator burned his body as he rolled on the ground, trying to extinguish the flames. Mario suffered third-degree burns on 80 percent of his body.

According to one of his treating doctors, living through this type of pain and injury is not easy. His flesh became scarred, his muscles became stiff, and pain racked his body. At the time, there was no rehabilitation for such an injury, and his father was told Mario would never walk again.

But Mario's dad refused to give up and accept such a hopeless prognosis. He would not allow his son to grow up disabled, immobile, and dependent on others. He decided to teach his son to walk in the small confines of their home. He created a wheelchair out of an old door and began a rigorous self-designed rehabilitation program for young Mario. He would not give in to despair. His son would walk again.

Over time, Mario was able to support his own weight and began to walk. He became even more active and was climbing fences and monkey bars again. He continued to improve and even played sports. He became a track star at DePaul Academy, played football and basketball, and began to be noticed by college scouts. Armed with an Italian-speaking priest, Notre Dame coach Elmer Leyden easily convinced the Tonelli family that Notre Dame was a better choice than the University of Southern California for Mario to begin his college football career. Mario would stay close to his midwestern roots and play football for Notre Dame.

His entry into Notre Dame football was not easy. He was assigned to the "hamburger squad" as a freshman. These were the players who were used to prepare the starters for games. Beaten up and bruised by training, Mario didn't quit. Instead, he worked harder—so hard that he earned a starting position on the squad his junior year.

In 1937, Mario became a legend at Notre Dame, winning a game over rival University of Southern California with a touchdown. No one ever thought Mario would walk, let alone play

football at the college level. When Mario graduated from Notre
Dame, he wore his ring as a symbol of perseverance and hope. His
career at Notre Dame was a victory on and off the field. Shortly
after, the Chicago Cardinals of the National Football League offered him a professional contract to play on their team.

However, his professional football career was interrupted when
World War II broke out. Mario felt obligated to serve and joined
the military. Leaving a new wife behind, he became an artillery
sergeant for the US Army. The war took him far away from home
to the Bataan Peninsula on the main Philippine island of Luzon.
While he was stationed in that area, Pearl Harbor was attacked,
and Mario knew the fight of his life was about to begin.

Months later, the Japanese advanced south into Bataan. Eventually, Mario and others were captured by the Japanese during
what has been called the "Alamo of the Pacific" in Bataan. The
Japanese forced thousands of prisoners to march a sixty-six-mile
death march that many didn't survive. But beaten, enslaved, tor-
tured, and ravaged by malaria and an intestinal parasite, Mario
never gave in to hopelessness.

The Japanese soldiers eventually took everything, including
Mario's precious Notre Dame ring. But moments after the ring was
taken, a Japanese officer who spoke English told Mario that he had
watched the 1937 game in which Notre Dame had beaten USC. He,
the officer, had been educated at USC. He was so impressed by the
game and Mario's play that he returned the ring to Mario. Mario
kept the ring as a symbol of hope—which he desperately needed,
given the brutality that escalated after that moment of humanity.
For the next three years, Mario endured constant, brutal torture,
and his 200-pound body wasted away to 130 pounds.

After being moved from prison camp to prison camp, Mario
came to the final camp of his long journey. He was assigned a pris-
oner number—58, the same number of his Notre Dame football
jersey. Mario could hardly hold back the tears. Hope welled up.

He would make it home. And he did. The war ended, and he was finally free after years of torture.

The ravages of war on his body required two surgeries upon his return. His stomach and intestines had to be repaired. But Mario was familiar with unthinkable challenges and fought his way back to health. The owner of the Chicago Cardinals offered him a place back on the team. While Mario was still recovering from malaria and schistosomiasis, he fought his way back to the football field and played against the Green Bay Packers. He proved to himself and the world that hope should never be lost.

Mario did not continue to play professional football but instead entered a life of politics and raised a family. In 2003, he left this earth, leaving us with a story of inspiration. He was a humble man who decided never to give up. His is a story of courage, humility, perseverance, overcoming, and hope.[1] Let his story inspire you never to give up and to live beyond your pain.

Acknowledgments

Linda: First and foremost, I acknowledge my family. To Norm, who has put up with my absences due to early morning writing sessions, weekends on the computer, and evenings hidden away to write, your loving support and patience for the process is what made this book possible. You are deeply loved, and I thank you. I also appreciate my academic colleagues for their encouragement and support and those who continue to do research in the area of pain management, providing updates and scientific evidence to direct patient care and programs. Keep doing the good work!

James: To Jennifer and our four children, please know how grateful I am for the sacrifice and patience you offered in the process of writing this book. Your support, love, and encouragement made it all possible. You are so deeply loved. Thank you, and I promise not to bring the laptop to the pool anymore. Also, thank you to the many educators, mentors, colleagues, coworkers, patients, students, family, and friends who've taught and encouraged me over the years. Lastly, thank you, Dr. Linda Mintle, for the privilege of writing this book with you. I am so grateful for the opportunity.

Notes

Introduction: Pain—A Part of Our Lives

1. Institute of Medicine, *Relieving Pain in America: A Blueprint for Transforming Prevention, Care, Education, and Research* (Washington, DC: National Academies Press, 2011), accessed May 30, 2018, https://www.nap.edu/read/13172/chapter/2.

2. "NIH Analysis Shows Americans Are in Pain," National Center for Complementary and Integrative Health, August 11, 2015, https://nccih.nih.gov/news/press/08112015.

3. "AAPM Facts and Figures on Pain," American Academy of Pain Medicine, 2017, accessed May 30, 2018, http://biomotionlabs.com/wp-content/uploads/2011/09/AAPM-Facts-Figures-on-Pain.pdf.

4. Peter D. Hart Research Associates, "Americans Talk about Pain," Researchamerica.org, August 2003, http://www.researchamerica.org/sites/default/files/uploads/poll2003pain.pdf.

5. "Global Pain Management Market to Reach US$60 Billion by 2015, According to a New Report by Global Industry Analysts, Inc.," PRWeb, January 10, 2011, https://www.prweb.com/releases/2011/1/prweb8052240.htm.

6. Grover et al., "Sevoflurane and Analgesia," *British Journal of Anaesthesia* 98, no. 5, (April 2007): 692, https://doi.org/10.1093/bja/aem077.

Chapter 2 The Toll of Chronic Pain

1. Alison Hodgson, *The Pug List: A Ridiculous Little Dog, a Family Who Lost Everything, and How They All Found Their Way Home* (Grand Rapids: Zondervan, 2016).

2. Dr. Paul Brand and Philip Yancey, *The Gift of Pain* (Grand Rapids: Zondervan, 1993).

3. Brand and Yancey, *The Gift of Pain*, 188.

4. Hodgson, *The Pug List*, 95.

Chapter 3 Take Inventory to Rebuild the House

1. Sheera F. Lerman et al., "Longitudinal Associations Between Depression, Anxiety, Pain, and Pain-Related Disability in Chronic Pain Patients," *Psychosomatic Medicine* 77, no. 3 (2015): 333–41, doi:10.1097/psy.0000000000000158.

Chapter 4 When Pain Doesn't Stop

1. "Overview of Chronic Pain Treatment," American Chronic Pain Association, 2018, accessed September 20, 2018, https://www.theacpa.org/wp- content /uploads/2018/03/ACPA_Resource_Guide_2018-Final-v2.pdf.

2. John J. Bonica, "Important Clinical Aspects of Acute and Chronic Pain," in *Mechanisms of Pain and Analgesic Compounds*, eds. Roland F. Beers and Edward Graham Bassett (New York: Raven Press, 1979), 15–29.

3. K. P. Grichnik and F. M. Ferrante, "The Difference between Acute and Chronic Pain," *Mount Sinai Journal of Medicine* 58, no. 3 (May 1991): 217–20.

4. John J. Bonica et al., *The Management of Pain* (Philadelphia: Lea and Febiger, 1990).

5. F. Willard, J. Jerome, and M. Elkiss, "The Essence of Pain Lies Mainly in the Brain," in *Foundations of Osteopathic Medicine*, ed. Anthony G. Chila (Philadelphia: Wolters Kluwer Health/Lippincott Williams & Wilkins, 2011), 228–52.

6. James E. Crisson and Francis J. Keefe, "The Relationship of Locus of Control to Pain Coping Strategies and Psychological Distress in Chronic Pain Patients," *Pain* 35, no. 2 (November 1988): 147–54, doi:10.1016/0304-3959(88)90222-9; and Timothy C. Toomey et al., "Pain Locus of Control Scores in Chronic Pain Patients and Medical Clinic Patients with and without Pain," *Clinical Journal of Pain* 9, no. 4 (December 1993): 242–47, doi:10.1097/00002508-199312000-00004.

Chapter 5 The Five Most Common Types of Pain

1. Michael A. Seffinger and Raymond J. Hruby, *Evidence-Based Manual Medicine* (Philadelphia: Elsevier Saunders, 2007).

2. Mark W. Weatherall, "The Diagnosis and Treatment of Chronic Migraine," *Therapeutic Advances in Chronic Disease* 6, no. 3 (2015): 115–23, doi:10.1177/2040 622315579627.

3. Richard A. Deyo and James N. Weinstein, "Low Back Pain," *New England Journal of Medicine* 344, no. 5 (2001): 363–70, doi:10.1056/nejm200102013440508.

4. Seffinger and Hruby, *Evidence-Based Manual Medicine*, 83.

5. Nancy Julien et al., "Widespread Pain in Fibromyalgia Is Related to a Deficit of Endogenous Pain Inhibition," *Pain* 114, no. 1 (March 2005): 295–302, doi:10.1016 /j.pain.2004.12.032.

6. Gracely et al., "Functional Magnetic Resonance Imaging Evidence of Augmented Pain Processing in Fibromyalgia"; and Leslie J. Crofford, "The Hypothalamic–Pituitary–Adrenal Axis in the Pathogenesis of Rheumatic Diseases," *Endocrinology and Metabolism Clinics of North America* 31, no. 1 (March 2002): 1–13, doi:10.1016/s0889-8529(01)00004-4.

7. Mathilde H. Boisset-Pioro, John M. Esdaile, and Mary-Ann Fitzcharles, "Sexual and Physical Abuse in Women with Fibromyalgia Syndrome," *Arthritis*

& *Rheumatology* 38, no. 2, (February 1995): 235–41, https://doi.org/10.1002/art
.1780380212.

8. Leslie J. Crofford et al., "Basal Circadian and Pulsatile ACTH and Cortisol
Secretion in Patients with Fibromyalgia and/or Chronic Fatigue Syndrome," *Brain,
Behavior, and Immunity* 18, no. 4 (July 2004): 314–25, doi:10.1016/j.bbi.2003.12.011.

Chapter 6 The Opioid Epidemic and Chronic Pain

1. William L. White, *Slaying the Dragon: The History of Addiction Treatment
and Recovery in America* (Bloomington, IL: Chestnut Health Systems/Lighthouse
Institute, 1998), 112–13.

2. Barbara Allison-Bryan, MD, "Opioid Pain Management: From Practice to
Regulation and Back Again" (lecture, Richmond, VA, March 15, 2018).

3. Allison-Bryan, "Opioid Pain Management."

4. Abigail J. Herron and Timothy Brennan, *The ASAM Essentials of Addiction Medicine* (Philadelphia: Wolters Kluwer, 2015), chap. 1.

5. Herron and Brennan, *The ASAM Essentials of Addiction Medicine*, chap. 6.

6. Gery P. Guy Jr. et al., "Vital Signs: Changes in Opioid Prescribing in the
United States, 2006–2015," *Morbidity and Mortality Weekly Report* 66 (2017):
697–704, https://www.cdc.gov/mmwr/volumes/66/wr/mm6626a4.htm.

7. "The Opioid Epidemic by the Numbers," US Department of Health and
Human Services, updated January 2019, https://www.hhs.gov/opioids/sites/de
fault/files/2019-01/opioids-infographic_1.pdf.

8. Lynn R. Webster, Beth Dove, and Steven D. Passik, *Avoiding Opioid Abuse
While Managing Pain: A Guide for Practitioners* (North Branch, MN: Sunrise
River Press, 2007), chap. 1.

9. Maureen V. Hill et al., "Wide Variation and Excessive Dosage of Opioid
Prescriptions for Common General Surgical Procedures," *Annals of Surgery* 265,
no. 4 (2017): 709, doi:10.1097/sla.0000000000001993.

10. "The 2013 National Survey on Drug Use and Health: Summary of National
Findings," report no. 14-4863, NSDUH series H-48 (Rockville, MD: Substance
Abuse and Mental Health Services Administration, 2014), 32.

11. Herron and Brennan, *The ASAM Essentials of Addiction Medicine*, chaps.
1 and 6.

12. Webster, Dove, and Passik, *Avoiding Opioid Abuse While Managing Pain*,
chap. 1.

13. "Opioid Abuse and Addiction," MedlinePlus, November 30, 2018, https://
medlineplus.gov/opioidabuseandaddiction.html.

14. American Psychiatric Association, *Diagnostic and Statistical Manual of
Mental Disorders: DSM-5* (Washington, DC: American Psychiatric Publishing,
2013), 540–41.

15. Howard Smith and Steven Passik, eds., *Pain and Chemical Dependency*
(New York: Oxford University Press; 2008), chap. 6; Herron and Brennan, *The
ASAM Essentials of Addiction Medicine*, chaps. 1 and 3.

16. "Medication and Counseling Treatment," Substance Abuse and Mental
Health Services Administration, accessed July 20, 2018, https://www.samhsa.gov
/medication-assisted-treatment/treatment.

Chapter 7 Not All in Your Head—Or Is It?

1. V. S. Ramachandran and Sandra Blakeslee, *Phantoms in the Brain: Probing the Mysteries of the Human Mind* (New York: William Morrow, 1999), 44.

2. Choong-Wan Woo et al., "Distinct Brain Systems Mediate the Effects of Nociceptive Input and Self-Regulation on Pain," *PLoS Biology* 13, no. 1 (2015): doi:10.1371/journal.pbio.1002036.

3. Olga Pollatos, Jürgen Füstös, and Hugo D. Critchley, "On the Generalised Embodiment of Pain: How Interoceptive Sensitivity Modulates Cutaneous Pain Perception," *Pain* 153, no. 8 (August 2012): 1680–86, doi:10.1016/j.pain.2012.04.030.

Chapter 8 Stress and Pain

1. Katarina Dedovic et al., "The Brain and the Stress Axis: The Neural Correlates of Cortisol Regulation in Response to Stress," *NeuroImage* 47, no. 3 (2009): 864–71, doi:10.1016/j.neuroimage.2009.05.074.

2. M. N. Baliki et al., "Chronic Pain and the Emotional Brain: Specific Brain Activity Associated with Spontaneous Fluctuations of Intensity of Chronic Back Pain," *Journal of Neuroscience* 26, no. 47 (2006): 12165–73, doi:10.1523/jneurosci.3576-06.2006.

3. Jessica K. Alexander et al., "Stress Exacerbates Neuropathic Pain via Glucocorticoid and NMDA Receptor Activation," *Brain, Behavior, and Immunity* 23, no. 6 (2009): 851–60, doi:10.1016/j.bbi.2009.04.001.

4. Bruce S. McEwen, "Physiology and Neurobiology of Stress and Adaptation: Central Role of the Brain," *Physiological Reviews* 87, no. 3 (2007): 873–904, doi:10.1152/physrev.00041.2006.

5. Masafumi Morimoto et al., "Distribution of Glucocorticoid Receptor Immunoreactivity and MRNA in the Rat Brain: An Immunohistochemical and in Situ Hybridization Study," *Neuroscience Research* 26, no. 3 (1996): 235–69, doi:10.1016/s0168-0102(96)01105-4.

6. Etienne Vachon-Presseau et al., "The Stress Model of Chronic Pain: Evidence from Basal Cortisol and Hippocampal Structure and Function in Humans," *Brain* 136, no. 3 (2013): 815–27, doi:10.1093/brain/aws371.

7. Laura E. Simons, Igor Elman, and David Borsook, "Psychological Processing in Chronic Pain: A Neural Systems Approach," *Neuroscience & Biobehavioral Reviews* 39 (2014): 61–78, doi:10.1016/j.neubiorev.2013.12.006.

8. Edward Walker et al., "Psychosocial Factors in Fibromyalgia Compared with Rheumatoid Arthritis," *Psychosomatic Medicine* 59, no. 6 (1997): 572–77, doi:10.1097/00006842-199711000-00003; Jerome Schofferman et al., "Childhood Psychological Trauma and Chronic Refractory Low-Back Pain," *Clinical Journal of Pain* 9, no. 4 (1993): 260–65, doi:10.1097/00002508-199312000-00007; and Julia V. Domino and Joel D. Haber, "Prior Physical and Sexual Abuse in Women with Chronic Headache: Clinical Correlates," *Headache: The Journal of Head and Face Pain* 27, no. 6 (1987): 310–14, doi:10.1111/j.1526-4610.1987.hed2706310.x.

9. Ronald C. Kessler et al., "Prevalence, Severity, and Comorbidity of 12-Month DSM-IV Disorders in the National Comorbidity Survey Replication," *Archives of General Psychiatry* 62, no. 6 (2005): 617, doi:10.1001/archpsyc.62.6.617.

10. Jillian C. Shipherd et al., "A Preliminary Examination of Treatment for Posttraumatic Stress Disorder in Chronic Pain Patients: A Case Study," *Journal of Traumatic Stress* 16, no. 5 (2003): 451–57, doi:10.1023/a:1025754310462.

11. Chadi G. Abdallah and Paul Geha, "Chronic Pain and Chronic Stress: Two Sides of the Same Coin?" *Chronic Stress* 1 (2017): doi:10.1177/2470547017704763.

12. K. E. Hannibal and M. D. Bishop, "Chronic Stress, Cortisol Dysfunction, and Pain: A Psychoneuroendocrine Rationale for Stress Management in Pain Rehabilitation," *Physical Therapy* 94, no. 12 (2014): 1816–25, doi:10.2522/ptj .20130597.

Chapter 9 The Importance of Marginal Gains

1. "A Person in Pain Is Like a Car with Four Flat Tires," American Chronic Pain Association, 2013, video, https://www.theacpa.org/acpa-car-with-four-flat-tires/.

2. "Tour De France Victories by Nation 1903–2017, Statistic," Statista, 2017, accessed September 25, 2018, https://www.statista.com/statistics/268022/nations -with-the-most-overall-wins-in-the-tour-de-france/.

3. Mike Stavrou, "Who Is Dave Brailsford, Marginal Gains and His Take on Bradley Wiggins Controversy," *Sun*, November 19, 2017, https://www.thesun.co .uk/sport/4937952/who-dave-brailsford-team-sky-manager-marginal-gains-brad ley-wiggins/.

4. G. Scrivener, "What Chris Froome's Tour De France Win Tells Us about Top-Flight Business Success," *Forbes*, August 24, 2017, https://www.forbes.com /sites/johnkotter/2017/08/24/what-chris-froomes-tour-de-france-win-tells-us-ab out-top-flight-business-success/.

Chapter 10 Traditional Approaches to Pain Management

1. Garry G. Graham and Kieran F. Scott, "Mechanism of Action of Paracetamol," *American Journal of Therapeutics* 12, no. 1 (January/February 2005): 46–55, doi:10.1097/00045391-200501000-00008.

2. Courtney Krueger, "Ask the Expert: Do NSAIDs Cause More Deaths than Opioids?" *Practical Pain Management* 13, no. 10 (November/December 2013): https:// www.practicalpainmanagement.com/treatments/pharmacological/opioids /ask-expert-do-nsaids-cause-more-deaths-opioids.

3. Angel Lanas et al., "A Nationwide Study of Mortality Associated with Hospital Admission Due to Severe Gastrointestinal Events and Those Associated with Nonsteroidal Antiinflammatory Drug Use," *American Journal of Gastroenterology* 100, no. 8 (2005): 1685–93, doi:10.1111/j.1572-0241.2005.41833.x.

4. Christopher J. Derry, Sheena Derry, and R. Andrew Moore, "Single Dose Oral Ibuprofen Plus Paracetamol (Acetaminophen) for Acute Postoperative Pain," *Cochrane Database of Systematic Reviews*, no. 6 (2013): doi:10.1002/14651858 .cd010210.pub2.

5. Derry, Derry, and Moore, "Single Dose Oral Ibuprofen"; and Helen Gaskell et al., "Single Dose Oral Oxycodone and Oxycodone plus Paracetamol (Acetaminophen) for Acute Postoperative Pain in Adults," *Cochrane Database of Systematic Reviews*, no. 3 (2009): doi:10.1002/14651858.cd002763.pub2.

6. Tony Touray et al., "Muscle Relaxants for Non-specific Low-back Pain," *Cochrane Database of Systematic Reviews*, no. 2 (2003): doi:10.1002/14651858 .cd004252.

7. Stephen E. Abram, *Pain Medicine: The Requisites in Anesthesiology* (Philadelphia: Mosby / Elsevier, 2006); and Mark S. Wallace and Peter S. Staats, *Pain Medicine and Management: Just the Facts* (New York: McGraw-Hill, 2005).

8. Josimari M. Desantana, Valter J. Santana-Filho, and Kathleen A. Sluka, "Modulation Between High- and Low-Frequency Transcutaneous Electric Nerve Stimulation Delays the Development of Analgesic Tolerance in Arthritic Rats," *Archives of Physical Medicine and Rehabilitation* 89, no. 4 (2008): 754–60, doi:10.1016/j.apmr.2007.11.027.

Chapter 11 Change Your Structure, Change Your Pain

1. M. Seffinger, J. Sanchez, and M. Friax, "Acute Neck Pain," in *Foundations of Osteopathic Medicine*, ed. Anthony G. Chila, DO (Philadelphia: Wolters Kluwer Health / Lippincott Williams & Wilkins, 2011), 979–89.

2. Mark Cantieri, DO, "Legacies of Drs. Gordon Zink and B. A. TePoortan" (lecture, AAO Convocation, Dallas, TX, March 2018).

3. Gert Bronfort et al., "Efficacy of Spinal Manipulation and Mobilization for Low Back Pain and Neck Pain: A Systematic Review and Best Evidence Synthesis," *Spine Journal* 4, no. 3 (2004): 335–56, doi:10.1016/s1529-9430(03)00177-3; B. W. Koes, L. M. Bouter, and Maurits W. Van Tulder, "Conservative Treatment of Acute and Chronic Low Back Pain," in *Neck and Back Pain: The Scientific Evidence of Causes, Diagnosis, and Treatment*, ed. Alf L. Nachemson and Egon Jonsson (Philadelphia: Lippincott Williams & Wilkins, 2000), 271–304; Sally C. Morton et al., "Spinal Manipulative Therapy for Low Back Pain," *Annals of Internal Medicine* 138, no. 11 (2003): 871–81, doi:10.7326/0003-4819-138-11-200306030 -00008; Edzard Ernst and Elaine Harkness, "Spinal Manipulation: A Systematic Review of Sham-Controlled, Double-Blind, Randomized Clinical Trials," *Journal of Pain and Symptom Management* 22, no. 4 (October 2001): 879–89; Olav Frode Aure, Jens Hoel Nilsen, and Ottar Vasseljen, "Manual Therapy and Exercise Therapy in Patients with Chronic Low Back Pain," *Spine* 28, no. 6 (2003): 525–31, doi:10.1097/01.brs.0000049921.04200.a6; and Tracy Lucente et al., "A Comparison of Osteopathic Spinal Manipulation with Standard Care for Patients with Low Back Pain," *New England Journal of Medicine* 341, no. 19 (1999): 1426–31, doi:10.1056/nejm199911043411903.

4. Michael A. Seffinger and Raymond J. Hruby, *Evidence Based Manual Medicine* (Philadelphia: Elsevier Saunders, 2007), 83.

Chapter 12 Change Your Beliefs, Change Your Pain

1. Carol S. Dweck, *Mindset: The New Psychology of Success* (New York: Ballantine Books, 2016).

2. Marisol A. Hanley et al., "Pain Catastrophizing and Beliefs Predict Changes in Pain Interference and Psychological Functioning in Persons with Spinal Cord Injury," *Journal of Pain* 9, no. 9 (September 2008): 863–71, doi:10.1016/j.jpain .2008.04.008.

Chapter 13 Change Your Thoughts, Change Your Pain

1. J. Baxter et al., "The Role of Psychosocial Factors in the Pain Experience: The Relationship between Depression, Catastrophizing, and Chronic Pain," *Journal of Pain* 17, no. 4 (2016): S97–S98, doi:10.1016/j.jpain.2016.01.299.

2. Phillip J. Quartana, Claudia M. Campbell, and Robert R. Edwards, "Pain Catastrophizing: A Critical Review," *Expert Review of Neurotherapeutics* 9, no. 5 (2009): 745–58, doi:10.1586/ern.09.34.

3. Jennifer L. Boothby et al., "Catastrophizing and Perceived Partner Responses to Pain," *Pain* 109, no. 3 (June 2004): 500–506, doi:10.1016/s0304-3959(04)00122-8.

4. Irit Weissman-Fogel, Elliot Sprecher, and Dorit Pud, "Effects of Catastrophizing on Pain Perception and Pain Modulation," *Experimental Brain Research* 186, no. 1 (March 2007): 79–85, doi:10.1007/s00221-007-1206-7.

5. Michael J. L. Sullivan, Scott R. Bishop, and Jayne Pivik, "The Pain Catastrophizing Scale: Development and Validation," *Psychological Assessment* 7, no. 4 (1995): 524–32, doi:10.1037/1040-3590.7.4.524.

Chapter 14 Change Your Emotions, Change Your Pain

1. Randolph M. Nesse and Phoebe C. Ellsworth, "Evolution, Emotions, and Emotional Disorders," *American Psychologist* 64, no. 2 (February/March 2009): 129–39, doi:10.1037/a0013503.

2. Arne May, "Chronic Pain May Change the Structure of the Brain," *Pain* 137, no. 1 (July 2008): 7–15, doi:10.1016/j.pain.2008.02.034.

3. Katja Franke et al., "Estimating the Age of Healthy Subjects from T1-Weighted MRI Scans Using Kernel Methods: Exploring the Influence of Various Parameters," *NeuroImage* 50, no. 3 (April 15, 2010): 883–92, doi:10.1016/j.neuroimage.2010.01.005.

4. Rea Rodriguez-Raecke et al., "Brain Gray Matter Decrease in Chronic Pain Is the Consequence and Not the Cause of Pain," *Journal of Neuroscience*, November 4, 2009, http://www.jneurosci.org/content/29/44/13746.

5. David A. Seminowicz et al., "Cognitive-Behavioral Therapy Increases Prefrontal Cortex Gray Matter in Patients with Chronic Pain," *Journal of Pain* 14, no. 12 (December 2013): 1573–84, doi:10.1016/j.jpain.2013.07.020.

6. Steven J. Linton and Johan W. S. Vlaeyen, "Fear-Avoidance and Its Consequences in Chronic Musculoskeletal Pain: A State of the Art," *Pain* 85, no. 3 (April 1, 2000): 317–32, doi:10.1016/s0304-3959(99)00242-0.

7. Yoshiro Shiba, Andrea M. Santangelo, and Angela C. Roberts, "Beyond the Medial Regions of Prefrontal Cortex in the Regulation of Fear and Anxiety," *Frontiers in Systems Neuroscience* 10, no. 12 (February 2016): doi:10.3389/fnsys.2016.00012.

8. Theodore Isaac Rubin, *The Angry Book* (New York: Touchstone, 1998).

9. Robert M. Sapolsky, *Why Zebras Don't Get Ulcers: An Updated Guide to Stress, Stress-Related Diseases, and Coping* (New York: W. H. Freeman, 1998), 308.

10. Harald Breivik et al., "Survey of Chronic Pain in Europe: Prevalence, Impact on Daily Life, and Treatment," *European Journal of Pain* 10, no. 4 (May 2006): 287–333, doi:10.1016/j.ejpain.2005.06.009.

11. David A. Fishbain et al., "Chronic Pain-Associated Depression: Antecedent or Consequence of Chronic Pain? A Review," *Clinical Journal of Pain* 13, no. 2 (July 1997): 116–37, doi:10.1097/00002508-199706000-00006.

12. Madhukar H. Trivedi, MD, "The Link Between Depression and Physical Symptoms," *Primary Care Companion to the Journal of Clinical Psychiatry* 6, supp. 1 (2004): 12–16.

13. K. Kroenke et al., "Physical Symptoms in Primary Care: Predictors of Psychiatric Disorders and Functional Impairment," *Archives of Family Medicine* 3, no. 9 (October 1994): 774–79, doi:10.1001/archfami.3.9.774.

14. Maurice M. Ohayon and Alan F. Schatzberg, "Using Chronic Pain to Predict Depressive Morbidity in the General Population," *Archives of General Psychiatry* 60, no. 1 (January 2003): 39–47, doi:10.1001/archpsyc.60.1.39.

15. David A. Fishbain, "The Association of Chronic Pain and Suicide," *Seminars in Clinical Neuropsychiatry* 4, no. 3 (August 1999): 221–27.

16. E. S. Paykel et al., "Residual Symptoms after Partial Remission: An Important Outcome in Depression," *Psychological Medicine* 25, no. 6 (1995): 1171–80, doi:10.1017/s0033291700033146.

17. H. J. McQuay et al., "A Systematic Review of Antidepressants in Neuropathic Pain," *Pain* 68, nos. 2–3 (December 1996): 217–27, doi:10.1016/s0304-39 59(96)03140-5.

18. Alfons Schnitzler and Markus Ploner, "Neurophysiology and Functional Neuroanatomy of Pain Perception," *Journal of Clinical Neurophysiology* 17, no. 6 (December 1996): 217–27, doi:10.1016/s0304-3959(96)03140-5.

19. Ayse Devrim Basterzi et al., "IL-6 Levels Decrease with SSRI Treatment in Patients with Major Depression," *Human Psychopharmacology: Clinical and Experimental* 20, no. 7 (November 2005): 473–76, doi:10.1002/hup.717.

20. David A. Fishbain, "Evidence-Based Treatment Paradigms for Depressed Patients with Pain and Physical Symptoms," *Journal of Clinical Psychiatry* 70, no. 7 (July 1, 2009): S75–S82, doi:10.4088/jcp.8001tx4c.

21. Vladimir Skljarevski et al., "Efficacy and Safety of Duloxetine in Patients with Chronic Low Back Pain," *Spine* 35, no. 13 (June 2010): E578–85, doi:10.109 7/brs.0b013e3181d3cf15.

22. Amy S. Chappell et al., "Duloxetine, a Centrally Acting Analgesic, in the Treatment of Patients with Osteoarthritis Knee Pain: A 13-Week, Randomized, Placebo-Controlled Trial," *Pain* 146, no. 3 (December 5, 2009): 253–60, doi:10.1016/j.pain.2009.06.024.

Chapter 15 Change Your Relationships, Change Your Pain

1. Catherine Armitage, "Everything You Know about True Love and Pain Is Wrong," *Sydney Morning Herald*, February 18, 2016, https://www.smh.com.au /healthcare/everything-you-know-about-true-love-and-pain-is-wrong-20160128 -gmfzhc.html.

2. Armitage, "Everything You Know about True Love and Pain Is Wrong."

3. Tara Parker-Pope, "Love and Pain Relief," *New York Times*, October 13, 2010, https://well.blogs.nytimes.com/2010/10/13/love-and-pain-relief/.

4. Clifton B. Parker, "Stanford Research Explains Why Some People Have More Difficulty Recovering from Romantic Breakups," *Stanford News*, January 7, 2016, https://news.stanford.edu/2016/01/07/self-definition-breakups-010716/.

5. Tom Saariaho et al., "Early Maladaptive Schema Factors, Pain Intensity, Depressiveness and Pain Disability: An Analysis of Biopsychosocial Models of Pain," *Disability and Rehabilitation* 34, no. 14 (2011): 1192–201, doi:10.3109/09 638288.2011.638031.

6. Laura E. M. Leong, "Does Empathy Promote Emotion Regulation in the Context of Pain? An Experimental Investigation" (PhD diss., Wayne State University, 2013).

7. Raquel Ajo et al., "Opioids Increase Sexual Dysfunction in Patients with Non-Cancer Pain," *Journal of Sexual Medicine* 13, no. 9 (September 2016): 1377–86, doi:10.1016/j.jsxm.2016.07.003.

Chapter 16 Change Your Stress, Change Your Pain

1. A. M. Gaughan, R. H. Gracelyl, and R. Friedman, "Pain Perception following Regular Practice of Meditation, Progressive Muscle Relaxation and Sitting," *Pain* 41 (1990): doi:10.1016/0304-3959(90)92750-k.

2. Peter R. Giacobbi et al., "Guided Imagery for Arthritis and Other Rheumatic Diseases: A Systematic Review of Randomized Controlled Trials," *Pain Management Nursing* 16, no. 5 (October 2015): 792–803, doi:10.1016/j.pmn.2015 .01.003.

3. Giacobbi et al., "Guided Imagery for Arthritis and Other Rheumatic Diseases."

4. Frans G. Zitman, Philip Spinhoven, A. Corrie G. Linssen, and Richard van Dyck, "Hypnosis and Autogenic Training in the Treatment of Tension Headaches: A Two-Phase Constructive Design Study with Follow-Up," *Journal of Psychosomatic Research* 36, no. 3 (April 1992): 219–28, doi:10.1016/0022-3999(92)90086-h.

5. Friedhelm Stetter and Sirko Kupper, "Autogenic Training: A Meta-Analysis of Clinical Outcome Studies," *Applied Psychophysiology and Biofeedback* 27, no. 11 (April 2002): 45–98.

6. N. Kanji, "Autogenic Training," *Complementary Therapies in Medicine* 5, no. 3 (September 1997): 162–67, doi:10.1016/s0965-2299(97)80060-x.

7. Susan P. Buckelew et al., "Biofeedback/Relaxation Training and Exercise Interventions for Fibromyalgia: A Prospective Trial," *Arthritis Care & Research* 11, no. 3 (June 1998): 196–209, doi:10.1002/art.1790110307.

8. Gary Elkins, Mark P. Jensen, and David R. Patterson, "Hypnotherapy for the Management of Chronic Pain," *International Journal of Clinical and Experimental Hypnosis* 55, no. 3 (July 2007): 275–87, doi:10.1080/0020714070 1338621.

9. Viatchslav Wlassoff, "The Neurological Mechanisms Behind Hypnosis," BrainBlogger, January 9, 2016, http://brainblogger.com/2016/01/09/the-neuro logical-mechanisms-behind-hypnosis/.

10. Heidi Jiang et al., "Brain Activity and Functional Connectivity Associated with Hypnosis," *Cerebral Cortex* 27, no. 8 (July 2016): 4083–93, doi:10.1093 /cercor/bhw220.

11. J. L. Spira and D. Spiegel, "Hypnosis and Related Techniques in Pain Management in the Terminally Ill," in *Noninvasive Approaches to Pain Management*

in the Terminally Ill, ed. Dennis C. Turk and Caryn Feldman (New York: Haworth Press, 1992), 89–119.

12. Virginia Heffernan, "The Muddied Meaning of 'Mindfulness,'" *New York Times*, April 14, 2015, https://www.nytimes.com/2015/04/19/magazine/the-mud died-meaning-of-mindfulness.html.

13. Britta K. Hölzel et al., "Mindfulness Practice Leads to Increases in Regional Brain Gray Matter Density," *Psychiatry Research: Neuroimaging* 191, no. 1 (January 30, 2011): 36–43, doi:10.1016/j.pscychresns.2010.08.006.

14. Steven Rosenzweig et al., "Mindfulness-Based Stress Reduction for Chronic Pain Conditions: Variation in Treatment Outcomes and Role of Home Meditation Practice," *Journal of Psychosomatic Research* 68, no. 1 (January 2010): 29–36, doi:10.1016/j.jpsychores.2009.03.010.

15. Steven C. Hayes, Kirk D. Strosahl, and Kelly G. Wilson, *Acceptance and Commitment Therapy: The Process and Practice of Mindful Change*, 2nd ed. (New York: Guilford Press, 2012).

16. Heffernan, "The Muddied Meaning of 'Mindfulness.'"

17. John Piper, "What Do You Think about Contemplative Prayer?" Desiring God, May 22, 2010, https://www.desiringgod.org/interviews/what-do-you-think -about-contemplative-prayer.

18. Fernando Garzon and Kristy Ford, "Adapting Mindfulness for Conservative Christians," *Journal of Psychology and Christianity* 35, no. 3 (October 1, 2016): 263–68.

19. Kristy Ford and Fernando Garzon, "Research Note: A Randomized Investigation of Evangelical Christian Accommodative Mindfulness," *Spirituality in Clinical Practice* 4, no. 2 (2017): 92–99, doi:10.1037/scp0000137.

20. Ahmet Muhip Sanal and Selahattin Gorsev, "Psychological and Physiological Effects of Singing in a Choir," *Psychology of Music* 42, no. 3 (April 2013): 420–29, doi:10.1177/0305735613477181.

21. Mimi M. Y. Tse et al., "Humor Therapy: Relieving Chronic Pain and Enhancing Happiness for Older Adults," *Journal of Aging Research* 2010 (May 25, 2010): 1–9, doi:10.4061/2010/343574.

22. Norman Cousins, *Head First: The Biology of Hope* (New York: E. P. Dutton, 1989).

23. R. I. M. Dunbar et al., "Social Laughter Is Correlated with an Elevated Pain Threshold," *Proceedings of the Royal Society B: Biological Sciences* 279, no. 1731 (2011): 1161–67, doi:10.1098/rspb.2011.1373.

24. Mayara C. S. Santos et al., "Association Between Chronic Pain and Leisure Time Physical Activity and Sedentary Behavior in Schoolteachers," *Behavioral Medicine* 44, no. 4 (November 10, 2017): 335–43, doi:10.1080/08964289.2017.1384358.

Chapter 17 Change Your Lifestyle, Change Your Pain

1. "Using Alcohol to Relieve Your Pain: What Are the Risks?" National Institute on Alcohol Abuse and Alcoholism, July 2013, https://pubs.niaaa.nih.gov /publications/PainFactsheet/painFact.htm.

2. "Dietary Guidelines for Americans 2005," US Department of Health and Human Services, updated July 9, 2008, https://health.gov/dietaryguidelines/dga

2005/document/html/chapter9.htm?_ga=2.9185532.812991222.1544578610-690
7690.1544578610.

3. Molly T. Vogt et al., "Influence of Smoking on the Health Status of Spinal
Patients," *Spine* 27, no. 3 (February 2002): 313–19, doi:10.1097/00007632-2002
02010-00022.

4. John Ulrich et al., "Tobacco Smoking in Relation to Pain in a National
General Population Survey," *Preventive Medicine* 43, no. 6 (January 2007): 477–81,
doi:10.1016/j.ypmed.2006.07.005.

5. Akiko Okifuji and Bradford Hare, "The Association between Chronic Pain
and Obesity," *Journal of Pain Research* 8 (July 14, 2015): 399–408, doi:10.2147
/jpr.s55598.

6. Nicola Torrance et al., "Severe Chronic Pain Is Associated with Increased
10 Year Mortality: A Cohort Record Linkage Study," *European Journal of Pain*
14, no. 4 (September 2009): 380–86, doi:10.1016/j.ejpain.2009.07.006.

7. Okifuji and Hare, "The Association between Chronic Pain and Obesity."

8. Holli C. Hitt et al., "Comorbidity of Obesity and Pain in a General Population: Results from the Southern Pain Prevalence Study," *Journal of Pain* 8, no. 5
(May 2007): 430–36, doi:10.1016/j.jpain.2006.12.003.

9. Andrea Kane, "How Fat Affects Arthritis," Arthritis Foundation, accessed
September 28, 2018, https://www.arthritis.org/living-with-arthritis/comorbidit
ies/obesity-arthritis/fat-and-arthritis.php.

10. Jackie MacMullan, "How Moses Malone Mentored a Young Charles Barkley," ESPN, September 14, 2015, http://www.espn.com/nba/story/_/id/13650802
/nba-how-moses-malone-mentored-young-charles-barkley.

11. Jenna Fletcher, "Dehydration Headaches: Signs, Treatment, and Prevention," Medical News Today, May 19, 2017, https://www.medicalnewstoday.com
/articles/317511.php.

12. "How an Anti-Inflammatory Diet Can Relieve Pain as You Age," Health
Essentials from Cleveland Clinic, October 19, 2017, https://health.clevelandclin
ic.org/anti-inflammatory-diet-can-relieve-pain-age/.

13. "How to Ease Your Arthritis Pain with Simple Food Swaps," Health Essentials from Cleveland Clinic, May 23, 2018, https://health.clevelandclinic.org
/simple-food-swaps-to-ease-arthritis-pain/.

14. Marie-Louise van Wetten, Leo Pruimboom, and Margarethe M. Bosma-
den Boer, "Chronic Inflammatory Diseases Are Stimulated by Current Lifestyle:
How Diet, Stress Levels, and Medication Prevent Our Body from Recovering,"
Nutrition & Metabolism 9, no. 1 (2012): 32, doi:10.1186/1743-7075-9-32.

15. J. L. Reed and A. H. Ghodse, "Oral Glucose Tolerance and Hormonal
Response in Heroin-Dependent Males," *BMJ* 2, no. 5866 (June 9, 1973): 582–85,
doi:10.1136/bmj.2.5866.582.

16. Patrick H. Finan, Burel R. Goodin, and Michael T. Smith, "The Association of Sleep and Pain: An Update and a Path Forward," *Journal of Pain* 14, no.
12 (December 2013): 1539–52, doi:10.1016/j.jpain.2013.08.007.

17. Nicole K. Y. Tang, "Insomnia Co-Occurring with Chronic Pain: Clinical
Features, Interaction, Assessments and Possible Interventions," *British Journal of
Pain* 2, no. 1 (September 1, 2008): 2–7, doi:10.1177/204946370800200102.

18. H. Foo and Peggy Mason, "Brainstem Modulation of Pain during Sleep and Waking," *Sleep Medicine Reviews* 7, no. 2 (April 2003): 145–54, doi:10.1053 /smrv.2002.0224.

19. Christian Guilleminault, Michelle Cao, Herbert J. Yue, and Pawan Chawla, "Obstructive Sleep Apnea and Chronic Opioid Use," *Lung* 188, no. 6 (December 2010): 459–68, doi:10.1007/s00408-010-9254-3.

Chapter 18 The Importance of Exercise and Movement

1. Louise J. Geneen et al., "Physical Activity and Exercise for Chronic Pain in Adults: An Overview of Cochrane Reviews," *Cochrane Database of Systematic Reviews*, no. 4 (April 24, 2017), doi:10.1002/14651858.cd011279.pub2.

2. Geneen et al., "Physical Activity and Exercise for Chronic Pain in Adults."

3. Patrick H. Finan and Michael T. Smith, "The Comorbidity of Insomnia, Chronic Pain, and Depression: Dopamine as a Putative Mechanism," *Sleep Medicine Reviews* 17, no. 3 (June 2013): 173–83, doi:10.1016/j.smrv.2012.03.003.

4. John Mayer, Vert Mooney, and Simon Dagenais, "Evidence-Informed Management of Chronic Low Back Pain with Lumbar Extensor Strengthening Exercises," *Spine Journal* 8, no. 1 (January/February 2008): 96–113, doi:10.1016/j .spinee.2007.09.008.

5. Rajiv Malhotra, "A Hindu View of 'Christian Yoga,'" *Huffington Post*, May 25, 2011, https://www.huffingtonpost.com/rajiv-malhotra/hindu-view-of-christ ian-yoga_b_778501.html.

6. Antonino Patti et al., "Effects of Pilates Exercise Programs in People with Chronic Low Back Pain," *Medicine* 94, no. 4 (January 30, 2015): doi:10.1097 /md.0000000000000383.

7. Kara Mayer Robinson, "Pilates," WebMD, 2017, accessed August 11, 2018, https://www.webmd.com/fitness-exercise/a-z/what-is-pilates.

8. Chenchen Wang et al., "Effect of Tai Chi versus Aerobic Exercise for Fibromyalgia: Comparative Effectiveness Randomized Controlled Trial," *BMJ* 360, no. K851 (2018): doi:10.1136/bmj.k851.

Chapter 19 When You Need More Help

1. David Niv and Shulamith Kreitler, "Psychological Approaches to Treatment of Pain: Sensory, Affective, Cognitive, and Behavioral," in *The Handbook of Chronic Pain*, eds. Shulamith Kreitler et al., (New York: Nova Biomedical Books, 2007), chap. 7.

2. Julie Loebach Wetherell et al., "A Randomized, Controlled Trial of Acceptance and Commitment Therapy and Cognitive-Behavioral Therapy for Chronic Pain," *Pain* 152, no. 9 (September 2011): 2098–107, doi:10.1016/j.pain.2011.05.016.

3. Kevin E. Vowles and Lance M. McCracken, "Comparing the Role of Psychological Flexibility and Traditional Pain Management Coping Strategies in Chronic Pain Treatment Outcomes," *Behaviour Research and Therapy* 48, no. 2 (February 2010): 141–46, doi:10.1016/j.brat.2009.09.011.

4. Olga Gutiérrez et al., "Comparison between an Acceptance-Based and a Cognitive-Control-Based Protocol for Coping with Pain," *Behavior Therapy* 35, no. 4 (Autumn 2004): 767–83, doi:10.1016/s0005-7894(04)80019-4.

5. Monica Buhrman et al., "Guided Internet-Delivered Acceptance and Commitment Therapy for Chronic Pain Patients: A Randomized Controlled Trial," *Behaviour Research and Therapy* 51, no. 6 (June 2013): 307–15, doi:10.1016/j.brat.2013.02.010.

6. Lance M. McCracken and Chris Eccleston, "Coping or Acceptance: What to Do about Chronic Pain?" *Pain* 105, nos. 1–2 (September 2003): 197–204, doi:10.1016/s0304-3959(03)00202-1.

7. Christopher Eccleston, Amanda C de C Williams, and Stephen Morley, "Psychological Therapies for the Management of Chronic Pain (Excluding Headache) in Adults," *Cochrane Database of Systematic Reviews*, no. 11 (November 14, 2012): doi:10.1002/14651858.cd007407.pub2.

8. B. Blair Braden et al., "Brain and Behavior Changes Associated with an Abbreviated 4-Week Mindfulness-Based Stress Reduction Course in Back Pain Patients," *Brain and Behavior* 6, no. 3 (2016): doi:10.1002/brb3.443.

9. Steven Rosenzweig et al., "Mindfulness-Based Stress Reduction for Chronic Pain Conditions: Variation in Treatment Outcomes and Role of Home Meditation Practice," *Journal of Psychosomatic Research* 68, no. 1 (January 2010): 29–36, doi:10.1016/j.jpsychores.2009.03.010.

Chapter 20 Complementary and Alternative Approaches to Pain Management

1. Shu-Ming Wang, Zeev N. Kain, and Paul White, "Acupuncture Analgesia: I. The Scientific Basis," *Anesthesia & Analgesia* 106, no. 2 (March 2008): 602–10, doi:10.1213/01.ane.0000277493.42335.7b.

2. Takahiro Takano et al., "Traditional Acupuncture Triggers a Local Increase in Adenosine in Human Subjects," *Journal of Pain* 13, no. 12 (December 2012): 1215–23, doi:10.1016/j.jpain.2012.09.012.

3. Matias Vested Madsen, Peter C. Gotzsche, and Asbjorn Hrobjartsson, "Acupuncture Treatment for Pain: Systematic Review of Randomised Clinical Trials with Acupuncture, Placebo Acupuncture, and No Acupuncture Groups," *BMJ* 338 (January 28, 2009): doi:10.1136/bmj.a3115.

4. Steven Novella, "Why I Am Skeptical of Acupuncture," *NeuroLogica Blog*, August 25, 2008, https://theness.com/neurologicablog/index.php/why-i-am-skeptical-of-acupuncture/; and Bruce Pomeranz and Daryl Chiu, "Naloxone Blockade of Acupuncture Analgesia: Endorphin Implicated," *Life Sciences* 19, no. 11 (December 1, 1976): 1757–62, doi:10.1016/0024-3205(76)90084-9.

5. Takano et al., "Traditional Acupuncture."

6. Fang-Chia Chang et al., "The Central Serotonergic System Mediates the Analgesic Effect of Electroacupuncture on *Zusanli* (ST36) Acupoints," *Journal of Biomedical Science* 11, no. 2 (March 2004): 179–85, doi:10.1159/000076030.

7. Pomeranz and Chiu, "Naloxone Blockade of Acupuncture Analgesia"; and Sven V. Eriksson, Thomas Lundeberg, and Stefan Lundeberg, "Interaction of Diazepam and Naloxone on Acupuncture Induced Pain Relief," *American Journal of Chinese Medicine* 19, no. 1 (February 1991): 1–7, doi:10.1142/s0192415x91000028.

8. Eiji Sumiya and Kenji Kawakita, "Inhibitory Effects of Acupuncture Manipulation and Focal Electrical Stimulation of the Nucleus Submedius on a Viscerosomatic Reflex in Anesthetized Rats," *Japanese Journal of Physiology* 47, no. 1 (1997): 121–30, doi:10.2170/jjphysiol.47.121.

9. K. Linde et al., "Acupuncture for the Prevention of Episodic Migraine," *Cochrane Database of Systematic Reviews*, no. 6 (June 28, 2016): doi:10.1002 /14651858.CD001218.pub3.

10. K. Linde et al., "Acupuncture for the Prevention of Tension-Type Headache," *Cochrane Database of Systematic Reviews*, no. 4 (April 19, 2016): CD 007587, doi:10.1002/14651858.CD007587.pub2.

11. John C. Deare et al., "Acupuncture for Treating Fibromyalgia," *Cochrane Database of Systematic Reviews*, no. 5 (May 31, 2013): doi:10.1002/14651858. cd007070.pub2.

12. Matias Vested Madsen, Peter C. Gotzsche, and Asbjorn Hrobjartsson, "Acupuncture Treatment for Pain: Systematic Review of Randomised Clinical Trials with Acupuncture, Placebo Acupuncture, and No Acupuncture Groups," *BMJ* 338 (January 28, 2009): doi:10.1136/bmj.a3115.

13. David M. DeChellis and Megan Helen Cortazzo, "Regenerative Medicine in the Field of Pain Medicine: Prolotherapy, Platelet-Rich Plasma Therapy, and Stem Cell Therapy—Theory and Evidence," *Techniques in Regional Anesthesia and Pain Management* 15, no. 2 (2011): 74–80, doi:10.1053/j.trap.2011.05.002.

14. David Rabago et al., "Dextrose Prolotherapy for Knee Osteoarthritis: A Randomized Controlled Trial," *Annals of Family Medicine* 11, no. 3 (May/June 2013): 229–37, doi:10.1370/afm.1504.

15. Kenneth D. Reeves and Khatab Hassanein, "Randomized Prospective Double-Blind Placebo-Controlled Study of Dextrose Prolotherapy for Knee Osteoarthritis with or without ACL Laxity," *Alternative Therapies* 6, no. 2 (March 2000): 68–74, 77–80; and Richard Dumais et al., "Effect of Regenerative Injection Therapy on Function and Pain in Patients with Knee Osteoarthritis: A Randomized Crossover Study," *Pain Medicine* 13, no. 8 (July 2012): 990–99, doi:10.1111 /j.1526-4637.2012.01422.x.

16. Fadi Hassan et al., "The Effectiveness of Prolotherapy in Treating Knee Osteoarthritis in Adults: A Systematic Review," *British Medical Bulletin* 122, no. 1 (June 1, 2017): 91–108, doi:10.1093/bmb/ldx006.

17. Ross A. Hauser et al., "A Systematic Review of Dextrose Prolotherapy for Chronic Musculoskeletal Pain," *Clinical Medicine Insights: Arthritis and Musculoskeletal Disorders* 9 (July 7, 2016): 139–59, doi:10.4137/cmamd.s39160.

18. Simon Dagenais et al., "Prolotherapy Injections for Chronic Low-Back Pain," *Cochrane Database of Systematic Reviews*, no. 2 (2007): doi:10.1002/14 651858.cd004059.pub3.

19. DeChellis and Cortazzo, "Regenerative Medicine in the Field of Pain Medicine."

20. DeChellis and Cortazzo, "Regenerative Medicine in the Field of Pain Medicine."

21. Mark S. Cantieri, "Prolotherapy," Corrective Care, 2018, accessed September 18, 2018, https://www.correctivecare.com/prolotherapy.

22. Mohini Ranganathan and Deepak Cyril D'Souza, "Medical Marijuana: Is the Cart Before the Horse?" *JAMA* 313, no. 24 (2015): 2431–32, doi:10.1001/jama .2015.6407.

23. Kathleen Doheny, "Can Marijuana Be the Answer for Pain?" WebMD, April 20, 2018, https://www.webmd.com/a-to-z-guides/news/20180420/can-mari juana-be-the-answer-for-pain.

24. Mahmoud A. Elsohly and Desmond Slade, "Chemical Constituents of Marijuana: The Complex Mixture of Natural Cannabinoids," *Life Sciences* 78, no. 5 (2005): 539–48, doi:10.1016/j.lfs.2005.09.011.

25. Wei Xiong et al., "Cannabinoids Suppress Inflammatory and Neuropathic Pain by Targeting α3 Glycine Receptors," *Journal of Experimental Medicine* 209, no. 6 (2012): 1121–34, doi:10.1084/jem.20120242.

26. Louise Marston et al., "Non-Invasive Brain Stimulation Techniques for Chronic Pain," *Cochrane Database of Systematic Reviews*, no. 4 (April 13, 2018). doi:10.1002/14651858.cd008208.pub4.

27. Ranganathan and D'Souza, "Medical Marijuana."

28. Ranganathan and D'Souza, "Medical Marijuana."

29. Shannon M. Nugent et al., "The Effects of Cannabis among Adults with Chronic Pain and an Overview of General Harms," *Annals of Internal Medicine* 167, no. 5 (August 2017): 319–31, doi:10.7326/m17-0155.

30. Rajiv Radhakrishnan, Samuel T. Wilkinson, and Deepak Cyril D'Souza, "Gone to Pot: A Review of the Association between Cannabis and Psychosis," *Frontiers in Psychiatry* 5, no. 54 (May 2014): doi:10.3389/fpsyt.2014.00054.

31. Tiziana Rubino et al., "Adolescent Exposure to THC in Female Rats Disrupts Developmental Changes in the Prefrontal Cortex," *Neurobiology of Disease* 73 (January 2015): 60–69, doi:10.1016/j.nbd.2014.09.015.

32. Russell K. Portenoy et al., "Nabiximols for Opioid-Treated Cancer Patients with Poorly-Controlled Chronic Pain: A Randomized, Placebo-Controlled, Graded-Dose Trial," *Journal of Pain* 13, no. 5 (May 2012): 438–49, doi:10.1016/j .jpain.2012.01.003.

33. Nugent et al., "The Effects of Cannabis among Adults."

34. National Academies of Sciences, Engineering, and Medicine (NASEM), *The Health Effects of Cannabis and Cannabinoids: The Current State of Evidence and Recommendations for Research* (Washington, DC: National Academies Press, 2017).

35. NASEM, *The Health Effects of Cannabis and Cannabinoids*, 90.

36. Doheny, "Can Marijuana Be the Answer for Pain?"

37. Doheny, "Can Marijuana Be the Answer for Pain?"

38. Ranganathan and D'Souza, "Medical Marijuana."

39. Marston et al., "Non-Invasive Brain Stimulation Techniques for Chronic Pain."

40. Herta Flor, Martin Diers, and Niels Birbaumer, "Peripheral and Electrocortical Responses to Painful and Non-Painful Stimulation in Chronic Pain Patients, Tension Headache Patients and Healthy Controls," *Neuroscience Letters* 361, nos. 1–3 (2004): 147–50, doi:10.1016/j.neulet.2003.12.064.

41. Marston et al., "Non-Invasive Brain Stimulation Techniques for Chronic Pain."

42. Marston et al., "Non-Invasive Brain Stimulation Techniques for Chronic Pain."

Chapter 21 Develop a Positive Mind-Set

1. G. Lorimer Moseley and Johan W. S. Vlaeyen, "Beyond Nociception," *Pain* 156, no. 1 (January 2015): 35–38, doi:10.1016/j.pain.0000000000000014.
2. David S. Butler and G. Lorimer Moseley, *Explain Pain*, 2nd ed. (Adelaide, Australia: Noigroup, 2013), 78.
3. Moseley and Vlaeyen, "Beyond Nociception."
4. Sara B. Algoe and Baldwin M. Way, "Evidence for a Role of the Oxytocin System, Indexed by Genetic Variation In *CD38*, in the Social Bonding Effects of Expressed Gratitude," *Social Cognitive and Affective Neuroscience* 9, no. 12 (January 2014): 1855–61, doi:10.1093/scan/nst182.
5. Paul J. Mills et al., "The Role of Gratitude in Spiritual Well-Being in Asymptomatic Heart Failure Patients," *Spirituality in Clinical Practice* 2, no. 1 (March 2015): 5–17, doi:10.1037/scp0000050.
6. Alex M. Wood et al., "Gratitude Influences Sleep through the Mechanism of Pre-Sleep Cognitions," *Journal of Psychosomatic Research* 66, no. 1 (January 2009): 43–48, doi:10.1016/j.jpsychores.2008.09.002.
7. Mei Yee Ng and Wing Sze Wong, "The Differential Effects of Gratitude and Sleep on Psychological Distress in Patients with Chronic Pain," *Journal of Health Psychology* 18, no. 2 (March 2012): 263–71, doi:10.1177/1359105312439733.
8. Robert A. Emmons and Michael E. McCullough, "Counting Blessings versus Burdens: An Experimental Investigation of Gratitude and Subjective Well-Being in Daily Life," *Journal of Personality & Social Psychology* 84, no. 2 (2003): 377–89, doi:10.1037//0022-3514.84.2.377.
9. Alex M. Wood, Jeffrey J. Froh, and Adam W. A. Geraghty, "Gratitude and Well-Being: A Review and Theoretical Integration," *Clinical Psychology Review* 30, no. 7 (November 2010): 890–905, doi:10.1016/j.cpr.2010.03.005.
10. James W. Carson et al., "Forgiveness and Chronic Low Back Pain: A Preliminary Study Examining the Relationship of Forgiveness to Pain, Anger, and Psychological Distress," *Journal of Pain* 6, no. 2 (March 2005): 84–91, doi:10.1016/j.jpain.2004.10.012.
11. Everett L. Worthington, *Forgiveness and Reconciliation: Theory and Application* (London: Routledge, 2006).
12. Steven C. Hayes, *Acceptance and Commitment Therapy: Part of Systems of Psychotherapy Video Series* (Washington, DC: American Psychological Association, 2009), DVD.
13. Robert D. Enright and Richard P. Fitzgibbons, *Helping Clients Forgive: An Empirical Guide for Resolving Anger and Restoring Hope* (Washington, DC: American Psychological Association, 2011), 67.
14. Michael J. A. Wohl, Rebekah L. Wahkinney, and Lise DeShea, "Looking Within: Measuring State Self-Forgiveness and Its Relationship to Psychological Well-Being," *Canadian Journal of Behavioural Science / Revue Canadienne Des Sciences Du Comportement* 40, no. 1 (January 2008): 1–10, doi:10.1037/0008-4 00x.40.1.1.1.

Chapter 22 Make Meaning Out of Pain and Suffering

1. Marilyn Baetz and Rudy Cecil Bowen, "Chronic Pain and Fatigue: Associations with Religion and Spirituality," *Pain Research and Management* 13, no. 5 (November 2007): 383–88, doi:10.1155/2008/263751.

2. Ginny Dent Brant, "An Honest and Inspiring Interview with Joni Eareckson Tada," Sonoma Christian Home, December 30, 2014, https://sonomachristian home.com/2013/05/an-honest-and-inspiring-interview-with-joni-eareckson -tada/.

3. Philip Yancey, *Where Is God When It Hurts?* (Grand Rapids: Zondervan, 2001).

4. Peter Kreeft, *Making Sense Out of Suffering* (New York: Phoenix Press, 1987).

5. C. S. Lewis, *The Problem of Pain* (New York: HarperCollins, 2014), 91.

6. Dorothy L. Sayers, "The Greatest Drama Ever Staged," in *The Whimsical Christian: 18 Essays* (New York: Collier Books, 1987), 12.

7. Timothy Keller, *Walking with God through Pain and Suffering* (New York: Penguin Books, 2016).

8. Viktor E. Frankl, *Man's Search for Meaning* (New York: Pocket Books, 1984).

9. Blaise Pascal, "Prayer, to Ask of God the Proper Use of Sickness," *Minor Works*, trans. O. W. Wright, The Harvard Classics, vol. 48, part 3 (New York: P. F. Collier & Son, 1909–14), https://www.bartleby.com/48/3/2/.

10. David Porter, *The Practical Christianity of Malcolm Muggeridge* (Downers Grove, IL: InterVarsity, 1983).

11. Paul Tournier, *A Doctor's Casebook in the Light of the Bible*, trans. Edwin Hudson (New York: Harper & Brothers, 1954).

Epilogue: Never Give Up

1. John Pandolfino, MD, "Motts and Me: The Story of Mario 'Motts' Tonelli," Motts 58 Foundation, March 4, 2018, https://motts58foundationorg.wordpress .com/mario-motts-tonelli/.

Linda Mintle, PhD, is a seasoned academic in the field of psychology and health care and has served on the faculty of two medical schools. She received her PhD in urban health and clinical psychology from Old Dominion University and a master's degree in social work and a bachelor of arts degree in psychology and communications from Western Michigan University. She is a national speaker, blogger, radio host of the *Dr. Linda Mintle Show*, and bestselling author with twenty books currently published. With twenty-seven years of clinical practice as a therapist and coach, she is directing her current clinical and academic efforts toward the development of an interprofessional approach to pain management given the present opioid crisis and the need for nonpharmacological approaches to help people deal with chronic pain.

James W. Kribs, DO, is a practicing physician and a graduate of Michigan State University, where he earned both a bachelor of arts degree in economics and a doctor of osteopathic medicine. Board certified in neuromusculoskeletal medicine with a subspecialty in pain medicine, he has focused on osteopathic manipulative medicine, manual sports medicine, medical orthopedics, and interventional pain management. He has served on the academic faculty of two medical schools and is involved nationally in advancing osteopathic medicine curriculum initiatives. He lives in Virginia with his wife, Jennifer, and their four children.

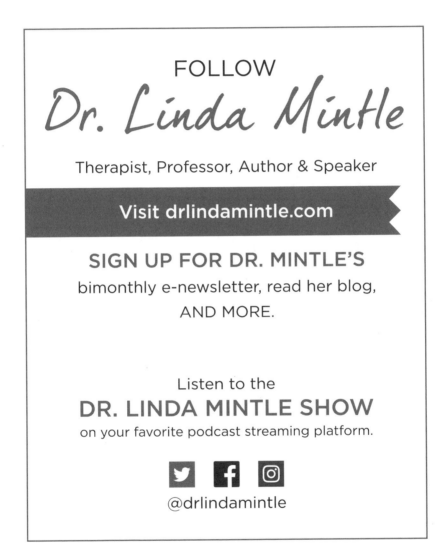

FOLLOW

Dr. Linda Mintle

Therapist, Professor, Author & Speaker

Visit drlindamintle.com

SIGN UP FOR DR. MINTLE'S
bimonthly e-newsletter, read her blog,
AND MORE.

Listen to the
DR. LINDA MINTLE SHOW
on your favorite podcast streaming platform.

@drlindamintle

FOLLOW

Dr. James W. Kribs, DO

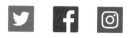

Visit drkribs.com

to read his blog and sign up for his newsletter.

@drjameswkribs